This book is to be returned on or before
the last date stamped below.

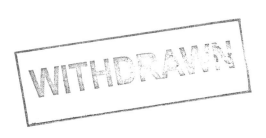

D1615624

HISTORY OF MEDICINE

DR BEHR ROOM
MACKENZIE HEALTHCARE LIBRARY
BURNLEY GENERAL HOSPITAL

A HISTORY OF
THE ROYAL COLLEGE
OF GENERAL PRACTITIONERS

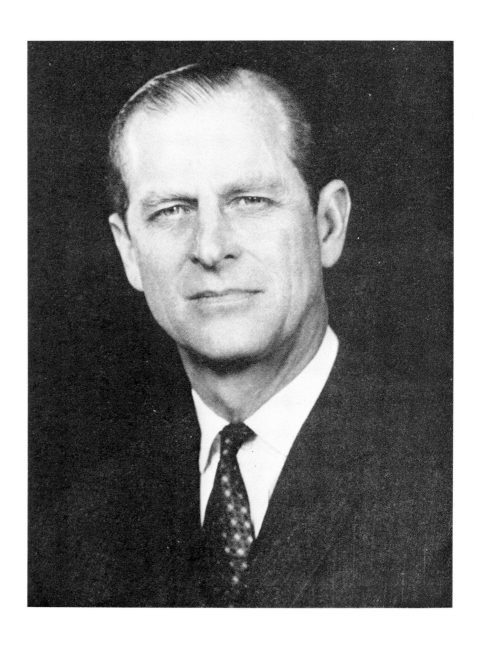

Frontispiece   HRH The Prince Philip, Duke of Edinburgh, KG, KT, OM, GBE, Patron of the College and President 1972

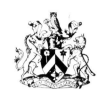

A HISTORY OF THE ROYAL COLLEGE OF GENERAL PRACTITIONERS

The First 25 Years

Edited by
John Fry
OBE, MD, FRCS, FRCGP

Lord Hunt of Fawley
CBE, DM (Oxon), FRCP, FRCS, FRCGP, FRACGP

and
R.J.F.H.Pinsent
OBE, MD, Hon.FRCGP

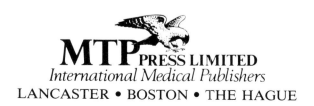

MTP PRESS LIMITED
International Medical Publishers
LANCASTER • BOSTON • THE HAGUE

Published in the UK and Europe by
MTP Press Limited
Falcon House
Lancaster, England

British Library Cataloguing in Publication Data

A History of the Royal College of General Practitioners.
1. Royal College of General Practitioners—History
I. Fry, John, 19--   II. Hunt of Fawley,
John Henderson Hunt, *Baron*   III. Pinsent,
R.J.F.H.
610′.6′042   R729.5.G4

ISBN 0-85200-495-8

Published in the USA by
MTP Press
A division of Kluwer Boston Inc
190 Old Derby Street
Hingham, MA 02043, USA

Library of Congress Cataloging in Publication Data
Main entry under title:

A History of the Royal College of General Practitioners.

   Bibliography: p.
   Includes index.
   1. Royal College of General Practitioners—History.
I. Fry, John, 1922- .   II. Hunt of Fawley, John
Henderson Hunt, Lord.   III. Pinsent, R.J.F.H. (Robert
John Francis Homfray) [DNLM: 1. Societies, Medical—
History—Great Britain. WB 1 FA1 R8]
R35.R473R68 1982   610′.6′041   82-18643
ISBN 0-85200-495-8

Phototypesetting by Georgia Origination, Liverpool
Printed by Butler & Tanner Ltd., Frome and London

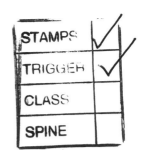

CONTENTS

vii

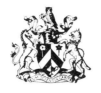

FOREWORD

John P. Horder, President, 1980–82

The first 30 years of the College have been an exciting experience for those most closely involved. Some have already passed on, but this account has been written soon enough for many of the actors to be historians. Future members of the College will be grateful to them for what they have written, as well as for what they did as a remarkably determined and harmonious team.

Students of twentieth century medicine in this country will also be grateful for a first-hand account of the development of an institution which has been closely associated with, and partly responsible for, important changes in medical care and education.

Those who read these pages may wonder how the builders of this young College could have found time to do much general practice. They did. The three editors of this history, which covers 25 years, and the general practitioner members of the Steering Committee all ran large practices, in which they worked very hard throughout that time. Most of their work for the College was done during off-duty hours, weekends and holidays. The College could not have developed as it did, had they not been personally concerned with the practical problems and needs of clinical medicine. This is also true of many of the contributors.

It is impossible to mention everyone who deserves credit. The editors hope that they may be forgiven for any serious omissions.

I want to thank both the editors and the contributors; in doing so, I know that I shall be joined by all those Fellows, Members and Associates whom for the time being I am proud to represent.

Especial thanks are due to Janet Smith, who typed all the drafts of the book with persistent goodwill. Very particular thanks are also due to Mr Robert Clark and others without whose generosity this book might never have been published.

JOHN P. HORDER, CBE, MD, FRCP, PRCGP

PROLOGUE

Sir Theodore Fox
Editor of The Lancet _1944–1964_

In 1952 general practice was in decline. Though many family doctors were working as well as ever, most were losing heart.

An Australian had been shocked by what he saw of British practice[1]; and two indigenous authorities had rejected the explanation that all its faults came from the National Health Service[2].

The truth was that, as the centre of gravity of Medicine shifted towards the hospital, practitioners had become less confident in their role. Some even accepted the view that they were second-class doctors, whose only important duty was to recognize serious conditions and refer these to their first-class colleagues.

This was quite wrong. Most medical care is given in the surgery or the home; and how it is given matters very much to very many. Nor is it easily given well. The efficient care of complex human beings in their natural state and natural habitat calls for more than a medical social worker or the subsidiary member of a specialist team.

To be good alike at primary care, continuing care, and terminal care demands high qualities. And in some ways the task grows harder as knowledge increases. The doctor in continuous personal charge of his patient – who may have diseases in several specialties – has to be very well informed if he is to know both what can be done and what _should_ be done.

Partly the College was founded to make a claim. If physicians, surgeons, and gynaecologists needed colleges, there was no less reason for general practitioners to have one. For their work – when done well – was of no less consequence. But, all too plainly, this work was not being done well enough: so a second object of the College was to examine the practitioner's changing functions and help him to perform them better. To this end the new body brought together a remarkable group of people. If their study of

xi

training, qualifications, postgraduate education and research had not proved so conspicuously useful, it would not have been copied and continued in similar colleges overseas.

Inevitably, some of the best doctors remain aloof, feeling no need for corporate recognition or support. But they too have gained because the status of general practice is rising. At a sad time in British Medicine, it is cheering to see that general practice is getting excellent recruits. Never again shall we hear those lamentable words: 'I'm only a GP'; for the labour in the College vineyard has not been in vain.

William A. R. Thomson

Editor of The Practitioner *1944–1972*

The tragedy of general practice in the early days of the National Health Service was that it lacked leadership. Those in authority in the planning and initiation of the Service – that is, the Ministry of Health and the Royal Colleges of Physicians, Surgeons and Obstetricians and Gynaecologists – knew comparatively little of family medicine. The British Medical Association, alas, adopted such an abrasive attitude toward the new service that it antagonized the Minister of Health responsible for the Service as it came into being.

The result was that the first quinquennium of the Service witnessed a demoralization of general practice that augured ill for the future. Political propaganda about 'free treatment' unleashed an utterly artificial demand that converted many a doctor's surgery into something resembling a bear garden. Unfortunately, both politicians and doctors were blinkered: the former by enthusiasm for party gain; the latter by equal enthusiasm for their own branch of the profession.

The concept of medicine as a healing art was overlooked, the co-operation essential to success became crude confrontation in the market-place, and what should have been a partnership in service to the community became a running battle in which some personalities assumed a disturbingly ominous influence. As a result the old men of general practice dreamt dreams of retirement, while the young ones saw visions of emigrating or transferring to some other branch of medicine.

It was as general practice reached this nadir that the concept of the College of General Practitioners was launched, based, in the words of the Report of the Steering Committee, on the belief that general practitioners are 'essential to the heart and soul of medicine' and, as I expressed it in *The Practitioner* at the time, that 'an active and progressive College of General Practitioners would safeguard the future of general practice as an integral part of the medical services of the country that offers a satisfying life's work to men of culture, understanding and integrity'[3].

This undoubtedly it has done. As in the pre-NHS days, general practice is now attracting those young men and women who have entered medicine in order to serve their fellow-citizens, who have the holistic outlook on life, and who have the innate curiosity of good naturalists such as Gilbert White, upon which they can build that intimate knowledge of the patient, his family and his environment, which is the basis of 'good general practice'. Largely as a result of its efforts over the last quarter of a century, the College has enabled general practice to find itself for many as the most satisfying branch of medicine – not a specialty, but the foundation stone of medical practice, and for this it deserves the thanks of all who look upon Medicine as the greatest profession of all.

Hugh Clegg

Editor of the British Medical Journal *1946–1965*

A leading article in the *British Medical Journal* on December 20 1952, discussing general practice in relation to the growth of specialization and special departments, suggested that general practitioners had been brought to a parting of the ways. It said:

> Unless something is done to reorient his training, undergraduate and graduate, to medicine as it is today – more exact and exacting, more of an applied science than an empirical art – the general practitioner risks becoming what Gerald Horner called 'a mere medical shopwalker'. It is clear that the moving spirits behind the College of General Practitioners have decided to meet the challenge of the times, and not too soon. Those who care for the welfare of medicine will thank them for their enterprise and foresight, and urge them forward along the path they have courageously taken[4].

References

1. Collings, J.S. (1950). General practice in England today. *Lancet,* **i,** 555–585
2. Lewis, R. and Maude, A. (1952). *Professional People.* London: Phoenix House Ltd.
3. College of General Practitioners (1953). Steering Committee's Report. *Practitioner,* **170,** Suppl.
4. *British Medical Journal* (1952). The College of General Practitioners, **ii,** 1344–1345

I
PAST ATTEMPTS TO FOUND A 'COLLEGE OF GENERAL PRACTITIONERS' ONE AND A HALF CENTURIES AGO

*John H. Hunt (*later *Lord Hunt of Fawley)*

Looking back, it is instructive and chastening to realize that more than a century ago a step to found a College of General Practitioners was carefully considered, and nearly taken. Then, as now, general practice was changing. There was much concern for its future, and for the academic welfare of family doctors; and in 1845 a widespread but unsuccessful attempt was made to preserve and improve their academic status by providing them with a college of their own[1].

In 1952, those who planned the new College had, at first, little (or no) knowledge of that previous endeavour[2]; and the difficulties they met throw into high relief the thoughtful opinions expressed by their predecessors in the remarkable and parallel previous effort which was revealed. There was a lesson of more than historical interest to be learned by reading the old reports, which I studied on many evenings in 1953 in the basement of the library of the Royal Society of Medicine.

To mention just a few. On June 9 1830, William Gaitskill (President of the Metropolitan Society of General Practitioners in Medicine and Surgery) wrote to the editor of *The Lancet*:

Various branches of the medical profession have colleges, charters and corporations, from which the general practitioner is either altogether excluded, or attached as an appendage only; he is not admitted to a participation in their councils, or to share in their honours; as a general practitioner, he belongs exclusively to no one branch, and is, therefore, virtually excluded from all. [*Lancet,* 1930, **ii,** 451]

1

In 1844, James Cole of Bewdley wrote:

> I will now tell you in what the remedy does really consist . . . which is so reasonable, so just, and so especially suited to the case. . . . The remedy I have to propose is the incorporation of the eighteen thousand Licentiates of the Hall into a 'Royal College of Apothecaries'. . . . By this simple means, we obtain what is wanting . . . a clearly defined, well and thoroughly educated body of medical practitioners . . . who . . . shall be in every way worthy of the respect of their colleagues and of public confidence. [*Provincial Medical and Surgical Journal,* 1844, **8**, 578]

George Webster of Dulwich had proposed the incorporation of general practitioners into a 'Royal College of Medicine and Surgery' [*Lancet,* 1844, **ii,** 241]. And George Ross of Kennington wrote:

> Dr Webster, in a letter you published last week, has declared the necessity of a College of General Practitioners. . . . The laws of the College of Surgeons are made for the Council and Fellows . . . let them retain their privileges, and enjoy the honours of their institution; but let the general practitioner have also his college – he has interests to support and a respectability to uphold; let him therefore possess the means of accomplishing these things. [*Lancet,* 1844, **ii, 318**]

The Worshipful Society of Apothecaries strongly supported this movement, and generously offered to withdraw its own interest in medical education in favour of the new College. The Provincial Medical and Surgical Association (the future British Medical Association), which had been founded by Charles Hastings in 1832, showed itself in favour. A meeting held on November 26 1844 (Dr Webster, President, in the chair) resolved:

> That the time has arrived when it has become imperatively necessary to adopt all legitimate means for the legal union of the General Practitioners of this kingdom into a distinct corporation. [*Lancet,* 1845, **i,** 133]

A National Association of General Practitioners in Medicine, Surgery and Midwifery was founded [*Lancet,* 1845, **i,** 127] for the purpose of petitioning for a Charter of Incorporation. At the first meeting of this Association (on 14 March 1845) about 1200 practitioners attended! *The Lancet* [1845, **i,** 326] said of this meeting:

The feeling of the meeting in favour of the representative principle was ardent, enthusiastic and unanimous.

Hopes ran high. But many serious constitutional errors were made in forming the permanent committee of this National Association. Bigoted, irresponsible, unforgivable blunders were made in its election, in its personnel (only one out of 60 resided more than ten miles from London), and in its actions. It refused to draw up a constitution or bye-laws, and it sent a draft Charter of Incorporation [Lancet, 1845, i, 191] to the Secretary of State, without submitting it first to a General Meeting [Lancet, 1845, i, 357-358]. All this aroused indignation, especially amongst country members; and the committee soon became detached and isolated, having forfeited the confidence not only of the National Association of General Practitioners [Lancet, 1845, ii, 391] but also of the whole profession.

Sir James Graham was drafting his Medical Bill for the better regulation of medical practice throughout the United Kingdom. It included the formation of a College of General Practitioners.

The editor of The Lancet – Thomas Wakley, MP, who was once described as 'The Father of Medical Reform' [Lancet, 1845, i, 420] – had written a leading article, and moved a resolution in Parliament urging that general practitioners had a right to demand that their College be founded with equal privileges and on equal terms with the existing Colleges [Lancet, 1845, i, 583-588].

A vast amount of argument took place, and the medical journals were full of it for months. In The Lancet this question of incorporating general practitioners into a College of their own, and the work of the committee formed for this purpose, was discussed in the leading article in no fewer than 41 of the 52 weekly issues in 1845. The hundred and more references to this subject in the medical journals at that time well repay careful study.

The medical profession as a whole, and Sir James Graham himself, were left perplexed and bewildered by all this argument and discussion, apart from their indignation and suspicion at the way the matter had been handled by the National Association's Committee. There was much disagreement and confusion, and the question of the foundation of a new college was postponed in favour of a reconciliation, and a closer and more honourable union, with the old.

R. M. S. McConaghey, ten years after the birth of our College, added some further interesting details about the introduction of the unsuccessful parliamentary Medical Bill, the object of which was to form a constitutional body to represent general practitioners (often called, in the past, 'surgeon-apothecaries') [Lancet, 1845, i, 415]. Great but unsuccessful efforts were made by Thomas Wakley, Sir James Graham,

George Webster and William Gaitskill towards this objective. Reform was in the air.

Further titles were suggested for the proposed organization – among them 'A College of General Practitioners in Medicine, Surgery and Midwifery', 'A Royal College of Medicine and Surgery', and 'A Royal College of General Practitioners of England'. The various Medical Parliamentary Bills were debated, amended, praised and supported, abused, committed and re-committed. The last, in 1854, was opposed both by the Royal College of Physicians and by the Royal College of Surgeons. People became weary of this endless controversy and, in the end, the Bill was shelved with the usual easy formula 'to be reintroduced next year'. But when that year came there was other work to be done, and the matter was dropped[3].

The possibility of combining all the Colleges into one all-embracing 'National College' was also in the air in 1845 – the equivalent of the modern suggestion to found an 'Academy of Medicine'[4] – but the difficulties were much the same as those we hear of today:

> The separate incorporation of the General Practitioners should be rendered unnecessary by the incorporation of the whole profession into one National College or Faculty of Medicine ... but the obstacles to the incorporation of the profession into one faculty, we are told, are insuperable, although the reasons for forming such an institution are unanswerable. [*Lancet*, 1845, i, 415]

We learnt a great deal from descriptions of this previous attempt: and I believe that we were able to avoid many pitfalls and blunders through the bitter experiences of our predecessors so many years ago, whose conceptions of a college ended in an unhappy and unfortunate miscarriage.

Acknowledgements

We are grateful to the editors of the many medical journals for permission to publish various paragraphs with suitable references in this book.

We are also very grateful to the College Librarian, Miss Margaret Hammond, and her staff for much help in compiling the references.

References

1. College of General Practitioners (1953). An attempt to found a College of General Practitioners 108 years ago. *First Annual Report Appendix I and II.*
2. Hunt, J. H. (1973). The Foundation of a College. *J. R. Coll. Gen. Practit.,* **23,** 5–19
3. McConaghey, R. M. S. (1972). Proposals to found a Royal College of General Practitioners in the nineteenth century. *J. R. Coll. Gen. Practit.,* **22,** 775–788
4. Sellors, T. H. *et al.* (1973). An Academy of Medicine. *Br. Med. J.,* **i,** 737

II
EVENTS LEADING UP TO THE FORMATION OF THE STEERING COMMITTEE

*John H. Hunt**

During the next hundred years (1850–1950), an academic body to represent general practitioners was again considered occasionally, but no other serious or combined attempts were made to follow up the matter. In 1944 Frank Gray[1] referred to it and, during the next seven years, several others spoke or wrote of a possible new college[2]. When the National Health Service was being planned many general practitioners felt lost without headquarters of their own, just as they had done more than a century before. After the introduction of the National Health Service in 1949, and the publication of the Collings Report[3] this need was appreciated more and more, and it was realized that there was a danger of general practitioners becoming isolated and of many of the standards and traditions of good general practice being lost. For too long, it was argued, had general practitioners carried on without headquarters, without academic leadership of their own, without much influence over undergraduate or postgraduate teaching, and without the status of their specialist colleagues. Specialists had rightly and properly built up for themselves their colleges, hospitals, diagnostic facilities, and many other things to help them in both the practical and academic aspects of their work and in research. General practitioners had muddled along, and time and time again they had found themselves left behind, edged out and even pushed out – as from certain (cottage) hospitals. Many practitioners felt that it was largely their own fault that they were in these difficulties. They had never organized themselves, and they had no one of the standing of the executive of the Royal Colleges to put forward their claims when big decisions had to be made. Some of them believed that a college of their own would help to put things right.

* *Geoffrey O. Barber, A. Talbot Rogers, Richard Scott* and others have all helped greatly with their recollections of the early days of the College

7

In this chapter we shall try to give some idea of the romance of the years 1951–2; of our feelings of helplessness at first, and of ignorance of how to set about the task of founding a new college; of our frustrations and disappointments when things went wrong; of anger when people laughed at us unkindly, or were unnecessarily rude (some of our acquaintances would not speak to us for a year or more); of our deep-felt gratitude for the encouragement and help we received from our true friends; and lastly of the excitement and feelings of fulfilment towards the end.

In 1936 Geoffrey Barber was talking about general practice to medical students at St Mary's Hospital – these were excellent lectures which were based on the contents of his doctor's bag, and some of which I attended; and in 1950 William Pickles (a general practitioner in Yorkshire) was lecturing up and down the country upon the epidemiological work of his country practice[4].

In 1947 the American Academy of General Practice was founded. This became, later, the American Academy of Family Physicians. In 1949 W. Edwards suggested a 'Royal College of General Practice'[5]; G. Ralston mentioned a 'Faculty of General Practice' in a letter to *The Lancet*, and signed himself FFGP[6]; and T. B. Layton, Guy's surgeon, suggested a 'Fourth Royal College'[7]. Then there was a talk by P. K. Murphy to the Chelsea and Fulham Division of the British Medical Association which was followed up by a letter from him in the *British Medical Journal* which was headed 'Royal College of General Practitioners'[8].

Geoffrey Barber discussed a possible new college with Sir Wilson Jameson one evening at Oxford, outside the Mitre Hotel, after a meeting of the Nuffield Provincial Hospitals Trust. After one of his lectures at St Mary's we dined together and talked about this. On another occasion soon afterwards, we dined with Aleck Bourne (gynaecologist to St Mary's Hospital) who gave us some useful ideas and encouragement.

In 1950, the Report of Sir Henry Cohen's Committee on *General Practice and the Training of the General Practitioner*[9] was timely. In June 1951 at the Annual General Meeting of the Medical Practitioners' Union a resolution was passed urging the development, without delay, of a 'College of General Medical Practice'. Bruce Cardew (the Union's general secretary at that time) was one of our most loyal and enthusiastic supporters for the next 20 years.

I was appointed to the Committee on General Practice of the Royal College of Physicians on April 26 1951. This met three times – in May, June and July. On one occasion a possible college for general practitioners was mentioned by me, but the suggestion was not well received and was not minuted. Professor J. M. Mackintosh (of the London School of Hygiene and Tropical Medicine) was also a member of that Committee and we had several private talks. We realized how disadvantageous it had been for general practitioners, when the National Health Service was being planned, not to have had behind them an academic body of their own.

In June 1951 George MacFeat (of Douglas, Lanarkshire) published a paper in the supplement of the *British Medical Journal* in which he suggested a Royal College of General Practitioners[10]. I wrote to him. Stephen Hadfield[11], who was travelling around Britain at that time collecting material for his Field Survey of General Practice, was talking soon afterwards to the Glasgow Division of the British Medical Association. He spoke to MacFeat about his paper; the latter pulled from his pocket some letters he had received and on the top one Hadfield recognized my handwriting. I had been a medical student with him.

As a direct result of this, I was invited to submit a memorandum to the General Practice Review Committee of the General Medical Services Committee of the BMA. Fraser Rose had previously approached the chairman of that committee about a possible college, and had also been invited to submit a memorandum which was dated 23 June. The request for those memoranda by this committee was, we believe, the first positive, active step taken towards the foundation of our College. I telephoned Fraser Rose the day before that committee met – the first time I had spoken to him.

We attended that historic meeting of the General Practice Review Committee in committee room A at BMA House at 1500 hours on October 3 1951. Fraser Rose sat on the right of the chairman (C. W. Walker from Cambridge) and I sat on the left. Rose spoke first to his excellent memorandum which set out very clearly what some people had been thinking that a new college might do, with several ideas of his own.

I told the meeting that I had drafted a letter which I had considered sending myself to the medical journals, the first eleven lines of which were almost the same as the third paragraph of my memorandum to the Committee; but, on consideration, I had thought that Fraser Rose should sign it too, because such a letter would carry more weight coming from two doctors with different kinds of practices and from widely different parts of the country.

A long, interesting, animated and, on the whole, favourable discussion about the two memoranda took place which lasted an hour and a half. Fourteen members of the Committee spoke. Annis Gillie (a general practitioner in London) was minuted as saying 'A College of General Practice may be a good idea so long as it does not demand more time from the general practitioner'. Little did we know what time-consuming work we were letting ourselves in for! Many of us owe a great debt to our patients, partners, and to our wives and families for all their forbearance, understanding, help and support during those past 25 years.

After the meeting, Fraser Rose, Geoffrey Barber and I met Sir Wilson Jameson who was waiting for us in the common room. We gave him our news and he told us how The Worshipful Society of Apothecaries, of which he was shortly to be Master, might be able to help.

Fraser Rose and I, having signed the letter, took it up to the office of the editor of the *British Medical Journal* and posted one to the editor of *The Lancet*. This letter appeared on October 13 1951[12]. Hugh Clegg and Theodore Fox, the editors, could not have been more helpful than they were then, or during all our College's formative years, in publishing our letters, papers, reports and notices.

Our letter read:

> There is a College of Physicians, a College of Surgeons, a College of Obstetricians and Gynaecologists, a College of Nursing, a College of Midwives, and a College of Veterinary Surgeons, all of them Royal Colleges; there is a College of Speech Therapists and a College of Physical Education; but there is no college or academic body to represent primarily the interests of the largest group of medical personnel in this country – the 20,000 general practitioners. Many practitioners sadly felt the lack of such a body when negotiations about the National Health Service were taking place . . .

Our letter went on to explain what was happening and ended:

> We are anxious to collect evidence upon this subject of a possible College of General Practice. If any of your readers have suggestions or comments to make, for or against this proposal, will they please communicate with us?

This letter attracted considerable notice, favourable and otherwise. We received much private correspondence about it; and many letters appeared in the *British Medical Journal* and in *The Lancet* during the next three months. Our two memoranda were published in the *British Medical Journal* a fortnight later[13,14].

I would like to put on record what an immeasurably important part Fraser Rose played at this time and during the later stages of the building up of our College. His friendship and wisdom, his generosity and unselfishness, his influence on the Council of the British Medical Association, his readiness always to help and advise, his quiet humour and good sense, and his judgement of character, were a very great help to us during many years.

Our training, fields of interest, practices, and connections were quite different, but in many ways they were complementary. I had several most interesting letters from him and a 16-page handwritten extract from his diary covering his college activities. I got to know him well, quickly, and we never had any significant disagreements; we met on a great number of occasions and were good friends. Fraser Rose had to travel a long way from Preston in Lancashire to be with us in London, and more than one illness made things particularly difficult for him. Sadly, he died on October 2 1972.

So much that so many people did forged links in the chain of events which culminated in the formation of our College. We should hear no more about who was responsible for founding it. *All* these people were responsible in different ways, including those who gave this matter so much thought more than a hundred years ago, those on the General Practice Review Committee and on our own Steering Committee. It has been a joint effort of many practitioners over several generations, helped by some consultants.

If George MacFeat had not written to the *British Medical Journal*, and Stephen Hadfield had not recognized my handwriting, I might not have met Fraser Rose, and would certainly not have submitted a memorandum to the General Practice Review Committee. Stephen Hadfield was the catalyst bringing Rose and me together. If Geoffrey Barber had not known Sir Wilson Jameson we might never have had the great help we did from the Worshipful Society of Apothecaries. Without Talbot Rogers, who was chairman of the General Medical Services Committee of the British Medical Association, our relations with the BMA, which were vital for our survival, might not have been nearly so friendly as they have been over the years; and we might even have had another name, for it was he who persuaded us to call ourselves 'The College of General Practitioners'. It was James Mackintosh who suggested that we should form a 'steering committee', a term with which we were not familiar. He said that it was just coming into use, and it proved most appropriate for what we wanted.

November and December 1951 were busy months. Mrs Geoffrey Evans and Ancrum Evans, old friends of mine, offered us the use of the ground floor of 7 Mansfield Street, and also, later, gave us the late Geoffrey Evans's library. I was invited to dinner by Angus Macrae (then Secretary of the BMA) and Stephen Hadfield to discuss further our possible relations with the BMA. On November 3 there was an encouraging editorial in the *British Medical Journal*[15].

On November 7 we wrote to Sir Heneage Ogilvie (Editor of *The Practitioner*) requesting help from his journal for our publications. Over the years he and his co-editor, William A. R. Thomson, were two of our keenest advisers and we owe a great deal to both. In a long and thoughtful reply Sir Heneage pointed out all the many difficulties which we faced, which made us more than a little despondent.

On November 15 I invited Fraser Rose and Ernest Busby, Clerk of The Worshipful Society of Apothecaries, to dinner; and six days later Fraser Rose and I visited that Society and were shown round. On November 17 we published a second letter in the medical journals asking for reports of any meetings at which a college was discussed[16].

On November 19 I read a short paper on the proposed college to the St Marylebone Division of the British Medical Association, which was published. On November 22 Sir Russell Brain (President of the Royal College of Physicians) invited me to dinner at the Athenaeum when we discussed in detail Sir Heneage's reply. Sir Russell thought that an autonomous joint faculty or academy of general practitioners within the three Royal Colleges would be better than a separate college.

What part was the new Section of General Practice of the Royal Society of Medicine going to take? Before our first letter appeared in the journals we had written to the President, Lord Webb-Johnson, among others, telling him what we were doing. He replied, 'I feel very strongly that to found a college would be a great mistake'. On November 25 I wrote to George Abercrombie (first President of the General Practice Section of that Society) suggesting a meeting there, so that we might discuss a possible college with several other general practitioners. But after careful and sympathetic consideration, and after consultation with the executive of the Royal Society of Medicine, this request was turned down because it was thought that such a meeting might be too 'political'. That was a disappointment because 'political' was the one thing we hoped we were *not*! Nevertheless, later on, seven members of the first two councils of that Section were on our Steering Committee, so there was close liaison between ourselves and the Society.

It was comparatively easy to suggest names for membership of the Steering Committee for which we wanted, at first, five practitioners and five consultants; but it was much harder to find a really good chairman. We were looking for a clever, independent-minded person who was outside the medical profession but who knew something about it, and who could influence other people. Michael Fletcher (Managing Director of *The Practitioner*) wrote to his brother-in-law, the Rt Hon Henry Willink (later Sir Henry Willink, Bt), Master of Magdalene College, Cambridge, outlining the position. Willink had been Minister of Health from 1943 to 1945, and had presented to the Coalition Parliament, in draft, the first White Paper on the National Health Service, in 1944.

On December 3 Willink replied that he would not give an immediate 'dusty answer' because, he said, 'I think that improvement of the conditions of general practice is of great and urgent importance'. But he pointed out that he lived in Cambridge: an hour's meeting in London took him away from his College for half a day; the Vice-chancellorship of the University was just over his horizon; the business we had in mind was particularly tricky and needed considerable knowledge of medical matters; and, as he had been a Tory MP from 1940 to 1948, that might be disadvantageous politically. Would not Sir Wilson Jameson (who had been Chief Medical Officer at the Ministry of Health) or Henry Brooke be better? I contacted the latter who was an old friend from Oxford days; he also was an MP and destined for the House of Lords later, but he said he was too busy with his parliamentary duties and with an impending London County Council election. So I wrote to Henry Willink on December 7 asking him to be our chairman. He was invited to dinner on December 18 but he suggested that, as he was already dining in London that evening, we should meet beforehand at the United University Club. This we did and had a long talk. In the end he said that he had the highest possible regard for Wilson Jameson's judgement and he would agree to be our chairman on one condition – 'That Wilson says I should'. Jameson pressed him strongly to accept our offer.

On December 8 there had been a critical editorial in *The Lancet* under the title 'Fragmentation or Integration'[17].

On December 12 Fraser Rose, Talbot Rogers and I visited 7 Mansfield

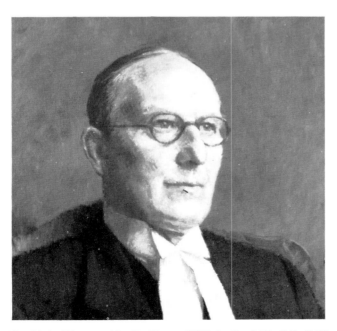

Plate 1   The Right Honourable Sir Henry Willink, Bt, MC, QC, DCL, MA

Street; we had dinner at The Bolivar restaurant opposite, during which we discussed many points about a possible college including a regional organization with faculties which, we all agreed, was essential.

In a few days' time I was able to write to Fraser Rose to tell him that, after several telephone calls, all ten whom we had invited to serve on the Steering Committee had accepted, and that Henry Willink *was* willing to be chairman. We cannot pay too high a tribute to Henry Willink and all he did to help us that year. He attended every one of our eight Steering Committee meetings, coming to London from Cambridge each time, often at great inconvenience to himself. As I said at the last meeting of the Committee,

> I am quite certain that no other person in this country could have helped us so much at a time when we wanted help so badly.

Later we made him our first Honorary Fellow and no one could ever deserve this honour more.

On December 29 a third letter[18] was sent to the journals announcing the formation and composition of our Steering Committee, and asking for constructive suggestions. The situation was now becoming critical.

A fortnight later, on January 11 1952, Sir Russell Brain wrote:

> Dear Hunt,
> In view of our talk and your recent letter in *The Lancet*, I think I ought to make it quite plain that this College, and I am sure I can here speak for the other two Colleges as well, would not be able to support in any way an organization which aimed at establishing another college or which it seemed to us might seek to do so at some future date. I can say this with confidence because this very point has just been settled by the three Royal Colleges jointly in connection with another matter. I want to make this plain now because, while, as you know, the three Royal Colleges would view sympathetically the establishment of a Joint Faculty of General Practice, I do not want those now considering the formation of some institution of general practice to go forward feeling that the three Royal Colleges would be likely to support an independent body without very stringent safeguards against its ever becoming a College.
> Yours sincerely, (signed) W. Russell Brain.

I replied:

> We may have some difficulty in persuading practitioners that you

are right in deciding that a Joint Faculty . . . will really serve them better, as their headquarters, than any other form of academic body. It will help us greatly at the first meeting of our Steering Committee if you could send us, please, during the next fortnight, your detailed reasons for this decision.

We were a little afraid of plans for integration with one or more of the Royal Colleges. Someone said once that integration was what the cat offered the canary! If you wanted the canary to sing it must be as an equal partner. *The Lancet* had a second somewhat unfavourable editorial on January 19[19].

On February 13 Sir Russell wrote again:

While I appreciate your difficulty I find it hard to know how I can help you further. I could not give details of what a Joint Faculty would imply, because I could not commit either this College or the others. Details would have to be worked out if the principle were accepted.

This meant that the 'Giants' (as Sir James Mackenzie had called his senior opponents some years before) were certainly going to oppose us. The task of rousing them to help us in a positive way was a thankless one from the beginning. They did not much wish to become involved, themselves, with the academic problems of general practitioners; and they did not really want anyone else to take steps, independently, towards a change. We were being asked to accept, in principle, a novel plan for a joint, but at the same time autonomous, faculty (which in itself seemed a contradiction in terms), about which no details were forthcoming, about which no one on either side knew anything, and which we almost certainly did not want anyway!

When we wrote to Lord Horder, asking whether he thought we should have a faculty or a college, he replied, 'I don't favour either!'

We were sure, then, that there was nothing for it but to call the 'Giants' to battle.

References

1. Gray, F. (1944). The general practitioner of the future. *Br. Med. J.,* **i,** Suppl. 121
2. College of General Practitioners (1953). *First Annual Report.* (London: CGP)
3. Collings, J. S. (1950). General practice in England today. *Lancet,* **i,** 555–585
4. Pickles, W. N. (1939). *Epidemiology in Country Practice.* (Bristol: J. Wright and Sons)
5. Edwards, W. (1949). In *Modern Trends in Public Health.* Massey, A. (ed) (London: Butterworths) p. 132

6. F.F.G.P. (Anticipatory). (1949). A Faculty of General Practice? *Lancet,* **i,** 372
7. Layton, T.B. (1949). A Faculty of General Practice. *Lancet,* **i,** 415
8. Murphy, P.K. (1949). 'Royal College of General Practitioners'. *Br. Med. J.,* **i,** Suppl. 124
9. Cohen Committee (1950). *General Practice and the Training of the General Practitioner.* (London: BMA)
10. MacFeat, G. (1951). The family doctor. *Br. Med. J.,* **ii,** Suppl. 1-3
11. Hadfield, S.J. (1953). A field survey of general practice 1951-52. *Br. Med. J.,* **ii,** 683-706
12. Rose, F.M. and Hunt, J.H. (1951). A College of General Practice. *Br. Med. J.,* **ii,** 908; *Lancet,* **ii,** 683
13. Hunt, J.H. (1951). A College of General Practice. *Br. Med. J.,* **ii,** Suppl. 175-176
14. Rose, F.M. (1951). General practice and special practice. *Br. Med. J.,* **ii,** Suppl. 173-175
15. *British Medical Journal* (1951). A college of general practice. **ii,** 1076-1077
16. Rose, F.M. and Hunt, J.H. (1951). College of General Practice. *Br. Med. J.,* **ii,** 1223; *Lancet,* **ii,** 943
17 *Lancet* (1951). Fragmentation or integration? **ii,** 1071
18. Rose, F.M. and Hunt, J.H. (1951). College of General Practice. *Br. Med. J.,* **ii,** 1582; *Lancet,* **ii,** 1226
19. *Lancet* (1952). Colleges and Faculties. **i,** 139

III
THE WORK OF THE STEERING COMMITTEE, AND THE BIRTH OF THE COLLEGE

Geoffrey O. Barber, John H. Hunt and A. Talbot Rogers

The 59 pages of minutes of the eight meetings of our Steering Committee are bound in the College's archives. At our first meeting at 7 Mansfield Street on February 28 1952 all but two of the five consultants and five general practitioners whom we had invited attended – Sir Wilson Jameson, Professor James Mackintosh (physicians), Professor Ian Aird (surgeon) and John Beattie (obstetrician and gynaecologist) – with four general-practitioner members – Geoffrey Barber, Talbot Rogers, Fraser Rose and John Hunt. The two who could not be there were Sir Heneage Ogilvie (surgeon), who was abroad, and our fifth general practitioner, J. MacLeod of Fraserburgh, who had accepted but had had to withdraw before the first meeting because of illness. Richard Scott of Edinburgh later took his place. Henry Willink, who also attended, was appointed Chairman.

John Hunt was elected honorary secretary and, as an introduction to the business, said, 'The object of the Steering Committee is to guide us towards an academic headquarters for general practitioners in an attempt to raise the standard and the status of general practice; to keep the better family doctors in general practice, to persuade other good ones to join them, and to encourage medical students to regard general practice as a branch of British medicine of which they could be justly proud'.

The letters from Sir Russell Brain were considered. Members of the Committee decided unanimously that they were opposed to the idea of a combined faculty. They thought that the Councils of the Royal Colleges were so busy with their own affairs that they would hardly have the time, or the inclination, to deal adequately with the academic problems of 20 000 general practitioners as well. We agreed that our organization should be autonomous, that the title 'College' would stimulate the imagination of

17

family doctors better than any other name, that we should remain academic, and not political, and that we should concern ourselves mainly with education and research.

We did not wish to wrangle with the Royal Colleges. Sir William Fletcher Shaw had told us how, before the College of Obstetricians and Gynaecologists was founded in 1929, the Royal Colleges of Surgeons and Physicians took them to court[1]. That was the last thing we wanted to happen to us.

On March 3 Willink wrote a charming letter to Sir Russell Brain:

> You will I hope forgive this unheralded letter . . . . Not unnaturally I am troubled by your letters to Hunt . . . in which you express the strongest possible opposition to the whole idea of an autonomous society for general practitioners. . . . You would I feel sure be willing to give me some guidance as to the objections felt by your-self and your fellow Presidents, and I wonder whether you would think it convenient to organize a meeting – possibly between the three Presidents and myself – when I could be shown the error of my ways!

Sir Russell invited him to lunch at the Royal College of Physicians with the other two Presidents – Sir Cecil Wakely and Dame Hilda Lloyd.

At the March meeting of our Steering Committee, Willink reported that he had had a frank, friendly and uninhibited discussion with the three Presidents. They were unanimously critical of the proposal to found a College of General Practitioners because they thought that this was merely an emotional reaction to the present state of general practice, that financing a new college would be difficult, that many practitioners would feel that it could not do much for them, and therefore they would not join, that it could not do its job properly if only a small proportion of general practitioners supported it, that the mass of general practitioners did not want further examinations or to pay examination fees, and that such a new college would very soon come up against opposition from the British Medical Association.

Some of this was quite correct and these were formidable arguments which would have quelled a lesser man than Willink. He was not, however, deterred. He asked the three Presidents what they suggested instead. They proposed, as before, an autonomous Joint Faculty, a new concept which Willink asked them to explain. He said that the phrase itself did not give a clear enough picture and that it would be difficult to ask practitioners to accept a mere phrase without any indication of what it meant.

Sir Russell replied that they would not work out a constitution only to have it rejected. The Presidents told Willink that they thought it would be disastrous if the College of General Practitioners went ahead against their opposition: they were opposed to it on principle.

Members of the Steering Committee were, however, all *for* a College of General Practitioners on principle, and the battle was now truly joined. As the Presidents could suggest no adequate alternative, it was agreed by our Committee that we should stand firm and not compromise. This was perhaps the most momentous decision in all our deliberations. And we still held the initiative.

At that second meeting, criteria for foundation membership were agreed and possible activities of the college discussed – undergraduate education and the part the College might play in the training of medical students and in vocational training after qualification, the development of trainee-assistant schemes, and the possibility of a new diploma later. James Mackenzie once wrote,

> There should be in every school of medicine one or more teachers who have been in general practice for ten to twenty years.

Three new general-practitioner members were appointed to the Steering Committee – David Hughes, James Simpson and R. J. F. H. Pinsent (usually known as 'Robin'). They all proved extremely useful members. James Simpson was Henry Willink's family doctor in Cambridge and acted as a link between the Steering Committee and its Chairman.

On April 9, with the Steering Committee's consent, one of us read a 'pulse-feeling' paper about the College to the South-west Essex Division of the British Medical Association[2]. Fraser Rose thought that it was 'entirely suitable for publication'. On April 18, we wrote to Sir Heneage Ogilvie saying,

> I feel that only about two per cent of practitioners in this country, so far, know what we are driving at and I hope that the publication of this paper will put the practitioners' case to the profession and present it in the right sort of way. Of those who have taken the trouble to put their ideas on paper and write either to the journals or to us privately, the proportion of those in favour to those against is over 50:1; so I feel sure that we have behind us the majority of doctors who have given thought to this matter.

But it was still not easy going. Some people laughed at us, others shunned us and some were downright rude, like the Fellow of the Royal College of Surgeons who met John Hunt in Wimpole Street and said, 'It's absolute nonsense, you might just as well found a college of ingrowing toe-nails!' To which he replied: 'That convinces me that a new college is really needed'. There was plenty of good-humoured banter too, like the cartoon in the *Birmingham Evening Despatch* showing a number of family doctors carrying their beds into an examination hall with a bystander saying, 'They're taking their bedside manner finals this week!'

At the May meeting of the Steering Committee it was agreed that yet another letter should be sent to the medical journals asking for small sub-scriptions to cover the expenses of the Steering Committee. A good response brought in more than £300. A practitioner in Hitchin, Sylvia Chapman, sent us £20. She later became the honorary assistant secretary of the Provisional Foundation Council and helped us greatly for many years. George Abercrombie, Richard Scott and J. B. Young of Belfast were to be invited to join the Steering Committee. The Honorary Secretary rang them up the next day but spoke to the wrong Dr Young, owing to a muddle over initials, and J. Campbell Young was invited by mistake. He accepted, and proved to be one of our most useful and successful members! He served on the College Council later for many years. When he died he generously remembered the College in his will.

Sir Francis Fraser (Director of the British Postgraduate Medical Federation of the University of London), who was an old friend, teacher and patient of John Hunt's, was on our side; and so was Sir Alexander Biggam, his opposite number in Scotland. They felt that while their organizations could arrange postgraduate courses, our proposed new college could, through its criteria for membership and in other ways, encourage general practitioners to attend them. We might also be able to advise on the content of these courses. Other senior members of our profession were sympathetic too, for which we were grateful: Sir Henry Cohen (later Lord Cohen of Birkenhead), Sir John Parkinson, Robert Platt (later Lord Platt), Harry Platt (later Sir Harry), James Spence (later Sir James), Arthur Porritt (later Lord Porritt), George Godber (later Sir George) and Charles Fleming among them; but they were not in power in the Royal Colleges at that time.

About then the Steering Committee had a long discussion on the part which general practitioners could play in research and how a college might be able to help in this. Sir Wilson Jameson told us that the Medical Research Council was willing to assist and had arranged a meeting to which four general-practitioner members of the Steering Committee were invited. We discussed a letter from George Swift.

> I wonder [it read] if you have ever come across the British Trust for
> Ornithology? They have done some very interesting research on

bird habits by choosing a bird of the year and sending a card to all members for the year. It occurred to me that perhaps a College of General Practitioners could do research in the same way.

Robin Pinsent described to the Steering Committee a helpful talk he had with the Regius Professor of Medicine at Oxford (Professor Arthur D. Gardiner) on this subject of general-practitioner research.

Believing that the Royal Colleges could not, or would not, produce definite plans for an alternative, we had the very difficult problem before us, now, of deciding just how we could form a college out of nothing. We had no organization on which to build, or which we could adapt, like the pathologists and the psychiatrists have had more recently, when they formed their colleges. We got little help from the history of the founding of the Law Society. Even the gynaecologists had their Gynaecological Visiting Society on which to make a start; and they had a very difficult task forming an incorporated company limited by guarantee, with a five-year gestation period and much trouble on the way, a court of enquiry, and with a considerable amount of internal quarrelling during that time.

On the advice of Henry Willink and another good friend of John Hunt's, Henry Benson (now Lord Benson) of Cooper Brothers (Chartered Accountants), we approached Sir Sam Brown of Linklaters and Paines (Solicitors), inviting him and his firm to help us over the complicated legal procedures inherent in founding a college. Sir Sam Brown and Mr John Mayo attended our fourth Steering Committee meeting when we discussed whether we should form our college as an unincorporated association, as an incorporated company limited by guarantee, or as an unlimited company.

They gave us excellent advice and, after a great deal of thought, we decided on the first. It had some drawbacks; but it was quick and we did not want to waste time or allow enthusiasm to dwindle, especially as the Danckwerts Award was to be distributed on January 1 1953 and we thought that practitioners might then feel more inclined to pay our entrance fee! We would not have to put a public notice in the press; we would not need the blessing of the profession, of the Royal Colleges, the Ministry of Health, nor of other Government Departments, nor even of the Board of Trade, although the last of these would have to agree to the name we chose. So long as our constitution was drawn up in the right way, our legal advisers told us that later on, when the value of our work was proven and we were generally accepted and financially sound, and when opposition was subsiding, we could change over, with little difficulty, to an incorporated company limited by guarantee, with a constitution almost the same as the one with which we started; and we could, later still, apply for a Royal Charter. This is just what happened.

On June 7 1952 a helpful editorial in *The Lancet*[3] was followed on June 27 by a most unfavourable one in the *Manchester Guardian*[4], under a heading 'FRCGP'; and another, nearly as bad, was in *The Times* the following day[5]. We remember that as a sad and worrying time when there was obviously much influential opposition, still, from the 'Giants' and others.

A personal letter was written to a number of influential doctors and others about the pulse-feeling paper which said,

> I am writing now to ask you (indeed to beg you) to withhold, please, any unrelenting or uncompromising disapproval or opposition to our plan for helping general practice, until all the evidence is collected . . . and until our Steering Committee's report is published. . . . Mr Henry Willink, the chairman of our Steering Committee, knows that I am writing this letter. He joins in my request and shares my hope.

Few of their replies were encouraging; but on the whole they were not *too* bad. Lord Horder wrote: 'My dear Hunt, Thank you. I will be good! Yours sincerely, Horder.'

The first draft of our Steering Committee's Report was presented to the Committee at its meeting in mid-September.

Number 7 Mansfield Street was soon to be sold, so on September 22 we wrote to Sir Wilson Jameson asking whether The Worshipful Society of Apothecaries would allow us to use its address for our first few years and its lovely Court Room and Hall for a few meetings. Their Court of Assistants, at a meeting on October 29 1952, very kindly acceded to this request – a wonderfully generous gesture on their part; and a great step forward for us, to be connected in this way with an established and well-known medical institution which had helped general practice greatly since early in the seventeenth century. In recognition of all this kindness and help, the College presented the Worshipful Society of Apothecaries in 1969 with a large silver Armada dish, which has been used regularly at their dinners since, inscribed round the rim:

> Presented by the Royal College of General Practitioners in gratitude for many kindnesses and for the hospitality so generously given to the college in its early days by the Master (Sir Wilson Jameson) and Wardens of the Worshipful Society of Apothecaries.

It was inscribed in the centre with the RCGP Owl over the Society's Rhinoceros, over the figures '1969'.

On October 31 the Honorary Secretary was asked to send 100 copies of his paper to Murray Stalker in Canada, who was planning to found a College of General Practice in that country.

The Honorary Secretary had written to John Mayo, our solicitor, on September 23 saying,

I feel fairly certain that the Steering Committee will take your advice (and that of Sir Sam Brown) to form an unincorporated body with a title of The College of General Practitioners.... Can you please tell me (1) whether you can arrange all this for us by January 1 1953, (2) whether there is any way in which the Royal Colleges can block us, or impede us before or after January 1, and (3) whether news of this move of ours is likely to leak out through the Board of Trade?

John Mayo replied favourably to all these questions.

In exactly two weeks he had not only prepared our Memorandum and Articles of Association, but he had obtained Counsel's opinion on them to make sure that we should be regarded as a charity, and that no other organization could say that we were poaching on its preserves; and copies had been printed for the Steering Committee to study and approve. He had drafted proposed bye-laws, too. He thought that we should plan for perhaps 500–1000 members during the first year of the College's life.

The Steering Committee had agreed that the headquarters of regional faculties of the College, at home and abroad, should be situated where possible in university cities. With the Committee's consent, John Hunt accepted an invitation to speak at a meeting of 18 postgraduate deans and directors of postgraduate education in Great Britain held in the Senate House of London University.

By that time many people thought that the foundation of our College was imminent, but very few knew just how or when it would appear. A leading article[6] in the *Postgraduate Medical Journal* said,

It is heartening to see that good seems about to rise from the depths to which general practice has been pushed in recent years. The reaction is likely to lead to the founding of a College of General Practitioners – a most salutary development for British Medicine, but one whose late appearance may well puzzle future medical historians.

Fraser Rose had spoken in Preston and in Blackpool about the proposed college; and John Hunt had done so also to the Wimbledon

23

Medical Society, to the Reigate, Redhill and Dorking Medical Society, and at the inaugural dinner of the Medical Practitioners' Union dining club. At these meetings very few people spoke against the idea. Sir Russell Brain was asked if any progress had been made with plans for a possible Joint Faculty of General Practice connected with one or more of the Royal Colleges, but he replied that they had done nothing further.

THE FOUNDATION OF THE COLLEGE

At the eighth and final meeting of the Steering Committee on November 19 1952 (less than nine months after it first met) our College was founded, when the Memorandum and Articles of Association were signed by its members, all of whom were present. Henry Willink remarked, 'It must have been just like this when they signed the American Constitution!'

This meeting was six weeks before the deadline of January 1 which we had set John Mayo. The College owes him a lasting debt for the magnificent work he did then, so quickly, and for everything he has done for us since. He and Ancrum Evans, our auditor, attended nearly all our annual general meetings and have advised us well whenever we have been in difficulty.

The Steering Committee's unanimous Report was signed on November 19 and published in the *British Medical Journal*[7] of December 20 1952, and as a supplement to *The Practitioner*[8] of January 1953, with full references to the discussions and correspondence mentioned above. In the committee's view, the evidence was overwhelming for the foundation as soon as possible of an academic body, with broad educational aims, to be the headquarters of general practitioners in Great Britain and to help and encourage them to maintain a high standard. The Committee had examined a great volume of evidence collected not only from all over the British Isles, but also from Canada, Australia, New Zealand and the United States of America.

Seven aspects of our problem had been studied by the Steering Committee: (1) the title, (2) functions, (3) criteria for foundation membership, (4) regional representation, (5) relations with other professional bodies, (6) accommodation and (7) finances. The conclusions of the report were as follows:

General practice is the oldest branch of medicine. Over 80 per cent of this country's illness is cared for by family doctors; and here as in Canada, Australia, New Zealand and the USA, it has been found that one of the most difficult tasks in medical administration and planning has been to find the proper role of the general practitioner in modern medicine. There is taking place now a worldwide

𝔐emorandum

AND

𝔄rticles of 𝔄ssociation

OF

THE COLLEGE OF GENERAL PRACTITIONERS

Formed the *19ᵗʰ* day of *November* 1952.

LINKLATERS & PAINES,
AUSTIN FRIARS HOUSE,
6 AUSTIN FRIARS,
LONDON, E.C.2.

S.L. 3147.

Plate 2   The cover and pages 6 and 7 of the original Memorandum and Articles of Association

6

WE, the several persons whose names and addresses are subscribed, are desirous of constituting and do hereby constitute a charitable association in pursuance of this Memorandum of Association.

NAMES, ADDRESSES AND DESCRIPTIONS OF SUBSCRIBERS

---

1. *[signature]* G. Abercrombie.
   76 Fitzjohn's Avenue,
   Hampstead, N.W.3.
   Medical Practitioner

Witness to the above signature :

[signature] Henry Willink
Magdalene College, Cambridge
Master of College.

2. *[signature]* Geoffrey Barber
   Road End.
   Dunmow. Essex
   Medical Practitioner

Witness to the above signature :

[signature] John Beattie.
147 Harley Street
W1.
Gynaecologist

Plate 2   (continued)

26

7

NAMES, ADDRESSES AND DESCRIPTIONS OF SUBSCRIBERS

3. David Hughes.
Green Parks
St Clears Carmarthen
Medical Practitioner

Witness to the above signature :

Wilson Jameson
8. Fordington Road
London N6
Physician

4. John Hunt.
54 Sloane St.
London S.W.1.
(Medical Practitioner)

Witness to the above signature :

Eileen Tarlton
Crispins Cottage
West Wittering, Sussex.
(Secretary)

5. [illegible] Pinsent
1 Hayfield Rd.
Handsworth
Birmingham
Medical Practitioner.

Witness to the above signature :

James M. Mackintosh
Chiltern Hill,
Chalfont St. Peter,
Bucks

Physician.

Plate 2 (continued)

reorientation of ideas about his capabilities and correct responsibilities, with a steadily growing conviction that general practice is
fundamentally as important as the specialties, and that it cannot be
controlled altogether by specialist organizations. General
practitioners have been in the past, and must be in the future, good
doctors practising medicine in their own right; they are essential to
the heart and soul of medicine. It is being increasingly realized that
this development and emancipation of general practice is not only a
question of professional pride and status but is an urgent economic
need – to keep patients out of hospitals whenever they can be
investigated and treated at home. Only by developing a higher
standard of general practice, and by making full use of properly
trained general practitioners (with access to hospital and laboratory
facilities), can the present overcrowding of outpatient departments
and excessive specialist consultations be avoided.

A golden opportunity now presents itself for general
practitioners to found an organization of their own, to watch over
their academic interests and their education. The Steering
Committee can find no evidence that any existing administrative
body in this country is doing now, or will be able to do in the
future, what practitioners require. Our evidence suggests that a new
college to lead general practitioners will help them more than will
any other organization, and that the influence of such a college for
the good of general practice cannot fail to be profound. We have
already had indications from all parts of the country that such a
college will have widespread support from practitioners themselves.
During the past twelve months, appeals have been made for an
alternative or better suggestion, but no better detailed proposal has
been put forward. The matter is urgent. In the words of *The
Lancet*, 'With the National Health Service still malleable, there is
much to be done now', and there is an immediate need for general
practitioners to establish for themselves an academic body that will
find its voice soon.

In this report we submit our considered proposals about the
new college, along lines which the majority of our correspondents
seem to desire. These are put forward in an attempt to construct a
framework for future development, in co-operation with existing
institutions. We realize that the final details of this college – its
exact name, the qualifications for its membership and fellowship,
its duties, its relations with other professional bodies, its premises,
finance etc, must be decided by general practitioners themselves,
and by no one else. The duty of the Steering Committee has been to

ensure that this matter was piloted safely up to the point where practitioners themselves could take the helm. . . . The Council and Foundation Members of the college will have a formidable task before them to develop an effective and permanent organization. Their path will inevitably be rough and beset with difficulties, and their progress may necessarily be slow. But they are assured of loyal and active support from many quarters; and we, the members of the Steering Committee, hope and believe that their ultimate achievements will be even beyond our expectations.

If the whole medical profession of Great Britain had been asked in 1952 to make a decision about founding the proposed new college, it seemed likely to the Steering Committee that years of interminable discussion would merely have ended in an indeterminate result.

George Ross, the first person so far as we know to mention in print the words 'College of General Practitioners' wrote[9] in *The Lancet* in 1844 that, in his opinion, rather than to wait 'standing by the riverside in expectation of some boon which the running waters may bear', it seemed better to 'launch its fortunes upon the current'. This is what the Steering Committee felt it right to do, a little more than a century later.

Thus 'The College of General Practitioners' was founded on November 19 1952, with a provisional constitution (Memorandum and Articles of Association and Bye-laws), with three criteria for foundation membership, and with a Provisional Foundation Council of ten general-practitioner members of the Steering Committee.

So our College was founded, but no one else knew this. The secret was well kept for several weeks longer – until the Steering Committee's Report was published. We could only sit back, then, and wait for our report to appear. That was one of the most anxious and exciting weeks of our lives.

References

1. Shaw, W. (1954). *Twenty-five Years*. (London: Churchill)
2. Hunt, J. H. (1952). A college of general practice. *Br. Med. J.,* i, Suppl. 335–339
3. *Lancet* (1952). Sequel to the Award. i, 1147–1148
4. *Manchester Guardian* (1952). FRCGP. 27 June, p. 6
5. *The Times* (1952). College of general practice. 28 June, p. 7
6. *Postgraduate Medical Journal* (1952). A college of general practitioners. **28,** 559
7. College of General Practitioners (1952). Report of the General Practice Steering Committee. *Br. Med. J.,* ii, 1321–1328
8. College of General Practitioners (1953). Report of the Steering Committee. *Practitioner,* **170,** Suppl.
9. Ross, G. (1844). On the necessity of incorporating the general practitioners. *Lancet,* ii, 318–319

IV
THE COLLEGE'S FIRST YEAR AND THE WORK OF
THE FOUNDATION COUNCIL

Geoffrey O. Barber, John H. Hunt, A. Talbot Rogers and Richard Scott

Our Steering Committee's Report was published on December 20 1952 as the first article in the *British Medical Journal*[1]. The news had been announced by the British Broadcasting Corporation in its morning bulletin the day before.

Immediate support, both welcoming and encouraging, was forthcoming from the editorial columns of the five leading medical journals in this country.

The *British Medical Journal's* comments[2] (leading article of December 20 1952) are quoted in the Prologue, above (page xiii).

The *Lancet* (leading article of December 20 1952) wrote[3]:

> ... it is believed that the very existence of a College will raise the status and enhance the prestige of the general practitioner amongst medical students, specialists and the public. We share that belief.... The backing of all of us is needed for what the founders of this new College rightly term 'their sincere attempt ... to improve the efficiency and good name of general practice'.

Its proprietors sent us a cheque for £100 because they felt that their first editor, Thomas Wakley, who was a general practitioner, would have wished them to give this support.

The *Practitioner* (leading article of January 1 1953) wrote[4]:

> The foundation of the College is an outstanding event in the history of British medicine.... It will bring fresh hope to many young

practitioners and a fresh incentive to the many medical students who see in general practice a career that will satisfy their highest ambitions.

It also published our report in full as a supplement to its January issue.

Medical Press (December 31 1952)[5] referred to the foundation of the College in its leading article as one of the great events of the past year.

Medical World (leading article, January 1953) wrote[6]:

> Medical men and women, whether general or special, must welcome the foundation of this new College. Its potentials are great. If wisely administered it could bring about vast changes for the good within a matter of years.

On January 2 we wrote to Willink to say that 52 lay newspapers had made favourable comments, one of them the *New York Times* that day!

A few people were angry; others thought that we had done something illegal, but Henry Willink and our admirable solicitors had seen to that. The favourable response was beyond our expectations. Telegrams and other messages of goodwill, and applications for membership, came flooding in. Ian Watson sent us a cheque for £100 to start a Foundation Endowment Fund, and other practitioners sent donations.

One of the most important personal letters which came to us was one from the secretary of the British Medical Association (Angus Macrae) which read,

> I need hardly say that I shall do anything I can to promote and maintain cordial and mutually helpful relations between the Association and the College.

This friendly attitude of the BMA was confirmed by a letter from its Council which read,

> The Council expressed itself as being entirely in sympathy with the objects of the College, and it noted with satisfaction that the College has no intention of competing with the Association in the medico-political field.

This was a unanimous expression, so Fraser Rose, who was present at the meeting, told us later.

Telegrams and letters of congratulation were received from many divisions of the British Medical Association, from many medical societies, from the President of the General Practice section of the Canadian Medical Association, the Director of the British Postgraduate Medical Federation of the University of London, the Master and Court of the Worshipful Society of Apothecaries, the deans of several medical schools, from many medical and surgical consultants, the Medical Committee of St Mary's Hospital, the Chairman of the Institute of Obstetrics and Gynaecology, and the Directors-General of the Royal Army Medical Service.

The Medical Protection Society sent the College a cheque for 100 guineas. Welcoming and congratulatory letters were also received from the General Medical Services Committee, the Private Practice Committee and the Science Committee of the BMA, the Medical Women's Federation (with the kind offer of a gift), from the British Medical Students' Association, the Institute of Hospital Almoners, the General Practitioners Society of New Zealand, the National Group of General Practitioners in South Africa, the Minister of Health for Tasmania, the Royal College of Midwives, the Pharmaceutical Society and the Scientific Film Association. Encouraging notices appeared from the General Secretary of the Medical Practitioners' Union and in the Bulletin of the Fellowship for Freedom in Medicine. The directors of Butterworth and Company (Medical Publishers) kindly offered the College a gold medal to be awarded annually. Letters from many doctors in support of the new College were published in the medical journals. Others, as was only to be expected, were critical; but these were few.

And lastly, and a somewhat surprising one, was from the President of the Royal College of Surgeons (Sir Cecil Wakely, Bt) which read, 'Best wishes for the happy start of the new College. I will always give all the support I can.'

Shortly before he died, Lord Horder invited one of us to visit him in his flat in Nottingham Place, where he sat in his red carpet slippers. He said he wanted us to know that although he had opposed us to start with, he now agreed with all that we were doing – a generous gesture on his part.

Sir Russell Brain also co-operated and this was surely a sign that these were great and good men with the welfare of our whole profession at heart. Their antagonism soon changed to friendship when they realized that we had achieved something that had been worth doing.

Applications for foundation membership (with certain criteria) were invited from January 1; some came in even before that date. By January 14, two weeks later, we were able to write to Fraser Rose to tell him that 1000 had joined as members (each paying an entrance fee of ten guineas), and 142 as associates. A few of them were consultants and specialists who were interested in the future of general practice or who had been in practice themselves in the past. By the end of six weeks the number had reached

1655, and £15 640 had been deposited in the bank.

Before the College was six months old, more than 2000 practitioners had joined, 130 of whom were from overseas. We never canvassed for members; to those who asked, 'What do we get out of joining your College?', we replied, 'The doctors we want are those who say "What can we give?" '

THE PROVISIONAL FOUNDATION COUNCIL

The first meeting of the Provisional Foundation Council, as we called it, was held a few minutes after the Steering Committee was dissolved. George Abercrombie was elected chairman: and what a superb chairman he was. Fraser Rose was vice-chairman, and John Hunt honorary secretary. Its other members were Geoffrey Barber, Talbot Rogers, Richard Scott, Campbell Young, J. D. Simpson, Robin Pinsent and David Hughes.

Arrangements were made for a great many papers to be printed – application forms for membership and associateship, memorandum and articles of association and bye-laws, bankers' order forms, receipt forms, writing paper and other items.

The objects of the Foundation Council were to lay the foundations of the College in the way that the Steering Committee had recommended, and to build up an adequate early membership so that it could present to the first Annual General Meeting, to be held 11 months later, a strong, firmly based and united young College which would be ready to take on the enormous amount of work which lay ahead.

At a second meeting, held on December 17, it was agreed that about 500 courtesy letters should be sent to the heads of all branches of the profession, at the time the Steering Committee's Report would appear, asking for their support and goodwill.

THE FOUNDATION COUNCIL

The Foundation Council was formed on February 18 1953 and was enlarged to 21 members by approaching all those general practitioners who had shown a particular interest in the Steering Committee's work – a good example of how our helpers almost chose themselves. From more than 500 names we picked 11, largely on a geographical basis to ensure fair regional representation; there was one woman, Annis Gillie. The Fates were certainly looking over our shoulders kindly when our small subcommittee of five (George Abercrombie, James Simpson, Richard Scott, David Hughes and John Hunt) prepared a short list. Without appreciating it fully at the time, we were deciding the future welfare of our College. Perhaps the rest of the 500 would have done as well as those we chose. They could hardly have done better.

The names of those 11 were: Annis Gillie, H. L. Glyn Hughes, Ian Watson, John Cottrell, George Swift, R. M. S. McConaghey, Douglas French, Guy Ollerenshaw, Ian Grant, John Henderson and Wilfrid Howells. All these played most important parts in the life of our College later on. Andrew Smith and J. F. Fleetwood were invited to join on April 5 1953.

A Finance and General Purposes Committee was elected by the Foundation Council on January 13 1953. H. L. Glyn Hughes was appointed honorary treasurer and Ancrum Evans auditor of the College.

On January 21 1953 three other committees were formed: an Under-graduate Education Committee, a Postgraduate Education and Regional Organization Committee and a Research Committee.

The Foundation Council met once a month in the Court Room of the Worshipful Society of Apothecaries, and many of these meetings were preceded by a meeting of one or more of its committees.

We were fortunate that we worked well together. The Foundation Council inherited from the Steering Committee a collective sense of purpose and the will and determination to achieve it which has remained with the College ever since. Naturally we have had differences of opinion, but quarrels and real acrimony have been at an absolute minimum. Those who founded our College, in 1952, were fortunate in discovering during the next two decades, better men and women than they themselves to carry on the work which they felt, so strongly, needed to be done for general practice. Throughout, it has been a most friendly team and some of our success has certainly been due to this.

In 1969 Sir George Godber (Chief Medical Officer of the Department of Health and Social Security) sent us a letter about our College:

I think the achievements of the last 17 years are without parallel in medical organizations in this country.

Two years later Sir Henry Willink, then aged 78, wrote:

I always feel that the foundation of the College was one of the very best projects with which I have been involved in my life.

During 1953 the Foundation Council appointed a Liaison Committee with the General Medical Services Committee of the British Medical Association, which has been very valuable over the years. An Undergraduate Committee issued a report presenting the case for the training of undergraduate medical students in those aspects of general practice best taught by general practitioners: it examined critically the existing arrangements for this, and discussed ways in which these might be extended and coordinated by enlisting the co-operation of the medical schools and the help of established practitioners. A Committee on Postgraduate Education issued a report in the medical journals on training a qualified doctor for a career in general practice, on continuing his education through his career, on encouraging a general practitioner to follow up a special bent, on providing a centre where they could meet and discuss their difficulties in their work and exchange views.

A Regional Council of the College was formed in Scotland and many pilot regional faculties at home and abroad were developed and their duties defined – 'to relieve the College Council of local responsibilities connected with activities of the College Council in the regions concerned'. Decisions were arrived at about the officers and members of faculty boards. The first criteria for membership and associateship of the College were decided upon. The entrance fee for foundation members was ten guineas and for associates one guinea. Members had to be on the Medical Register and to have spent 20 years in general practice or its equivalent, five years in general practice with an undertaking to accept postgraduate instruction, or five years in general practice with the possession of a higher postgraduate degree or diploma. Associateship of the College could be obtained by any qualified man or woman (general practitioner or consultant) who was interested in general practice.

When the house in Mansfield Street was sold by Geoffrey Evans early in 1953, the headquarters of the College moved to a room on the first floor at 54 Sloane Street SW1, above John Hunt's consulting rooms. This large room served as our headquarters for the next five years, where Sylvia Chapman (as assistant honorary secretary, assisted later by Mrs Eileen Phillips), did noble work.

The whole Foundation Council retired at the College's first general meeting on November 14 1953, which took place in the Great Hall at BMA House.

References

1. College of General Practitioners (1952). Report of the General Practice Steering Committee. *Br. Med. J.,* **ii,** 1321–1328
2. *British Medical Journal* (1952). The College of General Practitioners. **ii,** 1344–1345
3. *Lancet* (1952). College of General Practitioners. **ii,** 1211–1212
4. *Practitioner* (1953). College of General Practitioners. **170,** 1–3
5. *Medical Press* (1952). Medicine in 1952. **228,** 611–612
6. *Medical World* (1953). The College is formed. **78,** 46–48

V
PRESIDENTS AND CHAIRMEN OF COUNCIL OF THE COLLEGE DURING ITS FIRST TWENTY FIVE YEARS

John H. Hunt

John H. Hunt

PRESIDENTS

Before the first Annual General Meeting of the fully-formed College, on November 14 1954, a telegram of loyal greeting and humble duty was sent to Her Majesty The Queen. Her reply of thanks was received a few minutes before the meeting began.

At the meeting, William Pickles was installed as the first President of the College. He described this first meeting as 'a solemn and historic occasion'. There were few in the Great Hall of BMA House that afternoon who did not agree with him. The hall was full – more than 400 members and associates were present. Through the good offices of Ian Watson, His Excellency Monsieur Basile Mostras, the Greek Ambassador, presented the College with a gavel made from an ancient plane tree on the island of Cos.

The Foundation Council was re-elected as the first Council of the College with G. F. Abercrombie as chairman, F. M. Rose vice-chairman, H. L. Glyn Hughes as honorary treasurer and J. H. Hunt as honorary secretary.

The Foundation Council had decided that the executive director of the College should be the chairman of Council, with the President to represent the College at the many social and other functions to which we were invited, including major lectures with which the College was involved, which often took up much time and involved considerable travelling sometimes abroad, even as far as New Zealand. This division of responsibility has worked well:

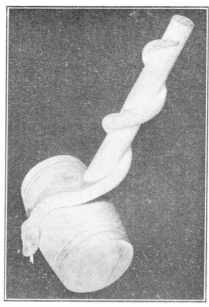

Plate 3 The College gavel, carved from the wood of a plane tree, on the island of Cos, under which Hippocrates was said to have taught

no one person could have done it all, especially if he was in active general practice. Both these offices would normally be held for three years.

Presidents:

W. N. Pickles	1953
I. D. Grant	1956
G. F. Abercrombie	1959
F. M. Rose	1962
Annis. C. Gillie	1964
J. H. Hunt	1967
G. I. Watson	1970
HRH The Prince Philip, Duke of Edinburgh	1972
P. S. Byrne	1973
E. V. Kuenssberg	1976

CHAIRMEN OF COUNCIL

As an indication of the College's development during its first 25 years we record a few highlights and special events which occurred during the terms of office of each chairman of council, written personally when possible.

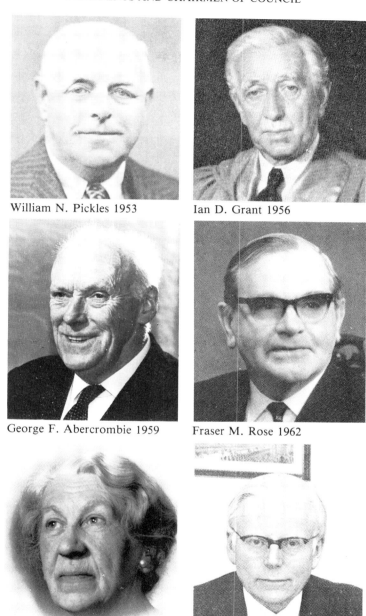

William N. Pickles 1953   Ian D. Grant 1956

George F. Abercrombie 1959   Fraser M. Rose 1962

Dame Annis C. Gillie 1964   John H. Hunt 1967

Plate 4   Presidents of the College 1953–1977

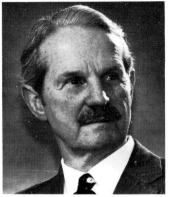

G. Ian Watson 1970

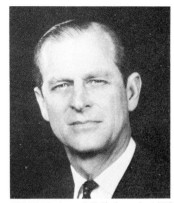

HRH Duke of Edinburgh 1972

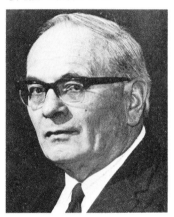

Patrick S. Byrne 1973

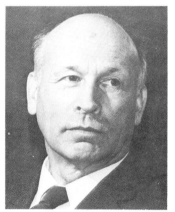

Ekke V. Kuenssberg 1976

Plate 4   (continued)

George F. Abercrombie

Chairman of Council 1953; *Died* September 25 1978

His term of office saw the formation of the College's 22 regional faculties in the British Isles, and it was agreed to publish a report from each of these every year (see Chapter VI). During his three years an extension throughout the College of the work of the teaching of general practice by general practitioners took place, and a report was published on the medical curriculum. The planning of postgraduate courses continued, and there was improved liaison between the College and universities and medical schools with the planning of departments of general practice in some of them. The research organization of the College was expanded, and different types of general-practitioner research explored (see Chapter XI). Three *Research Newsletters* were published. Full accounts of the College's progress, over the years, in educational matters – undergraduate, vocational and continuing education – will be found in Chapters VIII and IX.

The first Scottish Council was founded with J. M. Henderson as chairman. Criteria for membership and associateship and a possible examination were discussed. A Board of Censors was elected. Commander A. E. P. Doran was appointed lay secretary of the College. During George Abercrombie's term of office the first James Mackenzie Lecture was delivered by William Pickles on 'Epidemiology in Country Practice'. Subsequent Mackenzie lectures with references are listed in the Appendix.

At the Annual General Meeting in November 1956, the first Foundation Council Award 'for work of the highest merit in the realm of general practice' was made to R. J. Minnitt of Liverpool; and the first Butterworth Gold Medal was awarded to Donald Watt MacLean of Edinburgh for an essay on 'The Influence of Home Conditions during the First Five Years of Life'[1]. Geoffrey Barber delivered the second James Mackenzie Lecture on 'Medical Education and the General Practitioner', based on his lectures at St Mary's Hospital.

By the end of George Abercrombie's chairmanship of Council the number of members of the College had reached 2946, with 797 associates. Australian and New Zealand Councils of the College had been formed.

On the recommendation of an Awards Committee, the Rt Hon Sir Henry Willink and the five members of the Steering Committee who were consultants were appointed Honorary Fellows of the College.

George Abercrombie was the best Chairman of Council that the College could have had in its formative years. The Annual General Meeting on his retirement gave him a warm standing ovation; and a most moving vote of thanks was carried unanimously to one who had served the College so brilliantly during its first four years.

Fraser M. Rose

Chairman of Council 1956; *Died* October 2 1972

At the Fourth Annual General Meeting on November 17 1956, Ian Grant delivered the third James Mackenzie Lecture on 'Family Doctors: our Heritage and our Future'. On March 1 1957, John Hunt gave the Lloyd

41

Roberts Lecture in the University of Manchester on 'The Renaissance of General Practice'[2].

The New Zealand Council was founded on February 19 1957. A National Register of family doctors who were willing to take students was compiled. By the end of the year, 1200 names had been received, 450 of these were willing to have students to spend a week or more in their practices.

At the Fifth Annual General Meeting on November 16 1957, D. M. Hughes delivered the fourth James Mackenzie Lecture on 'Twenty-five Years in Country Practice' – a philosophical, poetical and amusing description of his early years of work in Wales, a 'peep into the country' when he joined a partner aged 83 in 'the good old days' which were not all good. He told of his hopes for the future of family doctors, and for the revitalizing influence of the College.

On July 1 1958, with 761 members and associates of our College in Australia, an autonomous Australian College of General Practitioners was formed. Many doctors remained members of both colleges for a while. A message to Australia from our President said, 'We hope that the ties which bound us so closely together during our formative years will still to a very large extent remain'.

In February 1958, the *Research Newsletter* became the *Journal of the College of General Practitioners*.

Through the generosity of Reginald Graham, the College moved its headquarters on March 11 1958, from 54 Sloane Street to 41 Cadogan Gardens, London SW3 (see Chapter XV).

The Medical Recording Service (see Chapter IX), under John and Valerie Graves, began work this year, helped by a generous grant from Smith, Kline and French Laboratories Ltd. It proved to be an enormous success.

At the Annual General Meeting on November 22 1958, further Honorary Fellows were elected, including Albert Schweitzer, OM. The fifth James Mackenzie Lecture was delivered by George Abercrombie on 'The Art of Consultation'. He made many wise comments, as,

It is really a good idea to regard the husband as one of the physical signs ... the family doctor must learn to manage not only the patient and relations and friends but, upon occasion, his specialist colleagues also; ... every consultation is a priceless opportunity of keeping up to date; [and] ... refreshing the confidence of patients.

Annis C. Gillie (later *Dame Annis Gillie*)

Chairman of Council 1959

The Seventh Annual General Meeting was held on November 21 1959. George Abercrombie was elected President. The sixth James Mackenzie Lecture was given by A. L. Vaughan Jones on 'The General Practitioner and Industrial Health'. He traced the growth of knowledge of occupational health since the time of Hippocrates.

During 1958 and 1959 much thought had been given to finding a permanent headquarters for the College. One possibility which was carefully considered was in Lincoln's Inn Fields, near the Royal College of Surgeons; another was on the Embankment; but there were reasons against both of these.

Some 300 members and associates attended the Eighth Annual General Meeting on November 19 1960. The election of Sir Harry Jephcott, who had done so much to help our appeal, as an Honorary Fellow was warmly received. The seventh James Mackenzie Lecture was given by Lindsey Batten (who was specially interested in the care of children) on 'The Medical Adviser'. Speaking about advice given to young mothers with young children and 'toddlers', he said,

> They, the toddlers, composed and performed their variations on a nursery theme ... they give innumerable performances year after year ... 'not use my pot', 'not eat my dinner', 'not sleep' ... it could even be shortened to 'not'; but so fertile are they in invention, so adept in the devices of augmentation, inversion and arrangement that every mother believes her particular little fiend to be playing a new tune. The medical adviser can get quite a long way by assuring her, with conviction, that the theme has the widest currency and that even the present variant has been heard before.

About young people, Dr Batten said,

> The medical adviser can – and I think he should – make the boy or girl know that they have in him an unshockable medical friend.

The College's achievement of Arms was finally settled after a long constructive debate covering two years (see Chapter XIX for a further description.)

The South African Council was appointed in 1961.

At the Annual General Meeting held on November 25 1961, a resolution of Council

That an examination in general practice be introduced as one of the criteria to be taken into account by the Board of Censors in considering applicants' requests for admission to membership of the College

was carried by 112 votes to 15.

Annis Gillie delivered the eighth James Mackenzie Lecture on 'James Mackenzie and General Practice Today'. As a thumbnail sketch of James Mackenzie her address can hardly be surpassed.

Mrs Glyn Hughes had been looking for a house to serve as permanent headquarters for our College. In July 1962 she found 14 Princes Gate, London SW7 – a large freehold property overlooking Hyde Park to the north and Ennismore Gardens to the south. It was ideal for our purposes and the College bought it quickly (see Chapter XV for further details and photograph.)

At the end of Annis Gillie's term of office the total membership of the College was 6311 (16 honorary fellows, 4041 members, 2221 associates and 33 corresponding associates from abroad). There were then 37 regional faculties of our College at home and overseas.

Kenneth McD. Foster

Chairman of Council 1962; *Died* October 28 1967

At the Annual General Meeting on November 24 1962, R. J. F. H. Pinsent delivered the ninth James Mackenzie Lecture on 'James Mackenzie and Research Tomorrow'. He gave a full description of the St Andrew's Institute for Clinical Research, which James Mackenzie founded in 1919. Sir James had said to the general practitioners of that city,

> You have the opportunity of seeing disease in the human subject in all its phases, of knowing the individuals before they become stricken . . . of seeing their surroundings and their mode of life. You are consulted at the first appearance of ill health and you see the patient through the whole course of his illness.

Robin Pinsent said that the flame which had been lit in the James Mackenzie Institute had recently burned low, to be fanned at many points at once as the concept of the College formed and took on substance.

The College moved into its new headquarters at 14 Princes Gate on January 2 1963. It had eight bedrooms and three flats for the use of members and associates, reservations being accepted for short periods (not

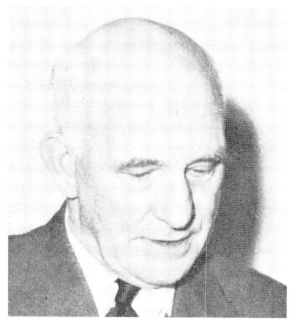

Plate 5   Kenneth McD. Foster 1962

more than 14 days at a time) and not for children under 12.

A handsome President's Badge in silver and enamel was presented by the Geigy Pharmaceutical Company Ltd to complete its generous gift of the President's Chain. It was made by Mr A. Styles of Garrard and Company Ltd (see Chapter XV).

At the Annual General Meeting on November 23 1963, John Henderson delivered the tenth James Mackenzie Lecture on 'Looking Back to Mackenzie'. He said,

> Look and listen.... Despite the ever-growing range of laboratory tests, the taking of a full and accurate case history remains the first and by far the most important single step in the systematic investigation of the majority of human ailments.
>
> It was Lord Cohen of Birkenhead who exhorted his students with the words 'Listen to the patient, gentlemen – he is *telling* you the diagnosis', to which John Henderson added 'and he is also mutely calling for help'.

Council learned with particular pleasure that Richard Scott had been appointed to the James Mackenzie Chair of Medicine in relation to General

Practice at the University of Edinburgh – the first chair of general practice in this country. The College's debt to him, as a member of the Steering Committee, and for his work in the field of undergraduate education, is very great.

Harry N. Levitt

Chairman of Council 1964

At the Annual General Meeting on November 21 1964, Professor Richard Scott's eleventh James Mackenzie Lecture was on 'Medicine in Society'. He pointed out how the present state of affairs in general practice in every country was the concern of nearly everyone and not only of family doctors themselves. He said,

> I welcome the increasing boldness of our own College in accepting the view that, while we are not, and never will be, a medical political organization, we must accept the challenge to produce yardsticks by which we can measure quality of care in general practice, and be more specific about the time, the tools and the training which are required.

Lady Churchill honoured the College by visiting headquarters on November 25 1964.

It was agreed by Council that all members of the College could belong to the College of General Practitioners' Club at 14 Princes Gate, London, SW7, where, on giving adequate notice, bed and breakfast could be obtained at reasonable rates and members could meet and entertain their friends and hire rooms for functions and meetings.

A court of examiners was appointed to hold a test of knowledge of the details of clinical medicine, and of all the other problems met with in general practice. The first examination was held on November 1 1965. Five candidates were successful (see Chapter X).

At the Annual General Meeting on November 20 1965, R. M. S. McConaghey's twelfth James Mackenzie Lecture was on 'Medical Practice in the Days of Mackenzie'. He wanted

> to try to place the young Mackenzie in his environment and to show the forces which drove him on to advance the study of cardiology in so unique a manner. . . . Our difficulties, great as they are, sometimes pale into significance when compared with those he had to overcome . . . without his tremendous drive, his patience, his

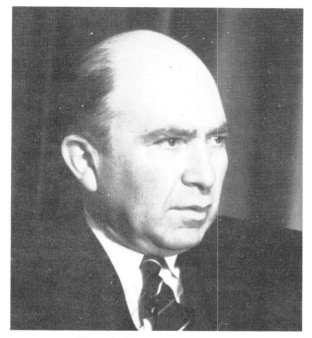

Plate 6   Harry N. Levitt 1964

perseverance, his buoyant personality and his humility, he could not have succeeded. . . . in the 1870s there were too many practitioners and, consequently, competition was keen, fees low, jealousy and ill-feeling very common and discontent rife. . . .

The College's Education Foundation Board began its work during this year.

On April 17 1967 a letter was received from the Home Office by H. N. Levitt which read:

I have the honour, by direction of the Home Secretary, to inform you that the Queen has been graciously pleased to command that the College of General Practitioners shall in future be known as 'The Royal College of General Practitioners'.

All our friends were delighted and a great many letters and messages of congratulations were received from individuals, and from national and international medical and paramedical bodies. While Council welcomed all

47

this goodwill shown toward our College it was very much aware not only of the honour but the increased responsibility which it carried.

At the Annual General Meeting held on November 19 1967, Ian Watson gave the thirteenth James Mackenzie Lecture on 'Learning and Teaching by Family Doctors'. Mackenzie, he said,

> exhibited in a high degree the persistence of all dedicated men who were unwilling to take 'don't know' for an answer.... He felt nothing of the mystery which now appears to surround the word 'research'... it means when you have made and recorded ten or a hundred observations, you should sometimes pause and look at them again, seeking to understand what they are trying to tell you.

At the end of Harry Levitt's term of office membership of the College had reached 7435 (24 honorary fellows, 5088 members, 2263 associates and 60 corresponding associates) – showing a steady increase each year.

George Swift

Chairman of Council 1967

Despite inevitable disappointments and frustrations this was a period of steady consolidation and development of policies already agreed. The Annual General Meeting on November 18 1967, formally acknowledged the College's Royal Prefix, and appointed its first Fellows. It agreed that entry to membership should be by examination in future. Many people, within and without the College, thought that on its fifteenth birthday it had firmly settled to join the establishment, and that it was in danger of becoming mediocre and stuffy.

Our task was to justify the resolution that had been passed: to identify a method of awarding Fellowships by which the title would be respected and sought after; to develop an examination which truly reflected the ability of successful candidates to perform as general practitioners; and as a corollary to identify and develop ways in which candidates could be educated for their vocation.

The highlight in developing the examination was the conference at the Royal College of Physicians in July 1968, when our ideas were tested and discussed by a distinguished gathering of doctors who were not general practitioners. By 1970 the examination seemed to be becoming generally accepted.

The Education Committee and its various subcommittees did an enormous amount of work, stimulated by the report of the Royal

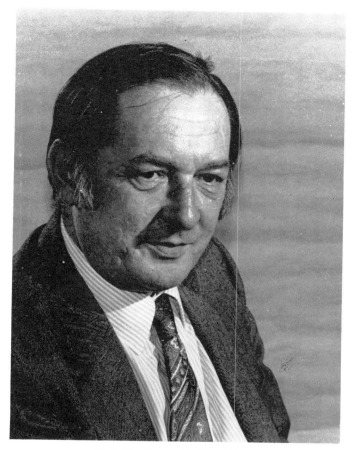

Plate 7   George Swift 1967

Commission on Medical Education which had favourably received the College's evidence. Its views on vocational training were accepted by the Conference of Local Medical Committees and by the Council of the British Medical Association. Important discussions were held with the General Medical Council which also accepted the College's ideas on training and, later, its Membership and Fellowship as registrable diplomas.

By 1970, due largely to the influence of the College, thirteen medical schools had departments of general practice, and postgraduate advisers were being appointed to set up vocational training organizations in the regions. Paradoxically, the College was losing its executive role in education and was having to redefine this.

1968 was a memorable year in the research field. The Ministry of Health agreed to finance the Records and Research Unit with a satellite study practice, and the Medical Research Council accepted our application for support for the Oral Contraception Study.

The development of relations with other bodies is an important part of a College's work. The Royal College of Physicians gave us great help in framing our Fellowship regulations, and in arranging a joint working party to study the place of the general practitioner in hospitals. Notable meetings were the Third International Conference of the World Organization of Colleges and Academies of General Practice held in Delhi in 1968, the visit of the Australian College at the Spring General Meeting in Aberdeen in 1970 and the joint meeting with the Canadian College in Toronto in the autumn of 1970.

At the Annual General Meeting in 1970 the first George Abercrombie Award was presented to R. M. S. McConaghey, for his editorial work.

Ekkè V. Kuenssberg

Chairman of Council 1970

The first full Council meeting in 1971 was a strange event. It was the first-ever Council meeting from which John Hunt was absent, and the last with Eileen Phillips as administrative secretary. She was followed by Commander James Wood, DSC, RN(Retd.). There was a report to Council that 50 candidates had taken the examination for membership, numbers which increased within a few years to 348 – continuing to rise to 580 per examination (see Chapter X). This was an indication of a new and different tempo that events were to take, as was the formation, and our representation on, the Central Council for Postgraduate Medical Education – probably our first inclusion as a member of a national medical organization of such fundamental importance. It was decided also to include a trainee as a member of College Council, and Council stimulated and then supported the National Conference of Trainees, which was to be held every two years.

Meetings took place with Dame Albertine Winner (Linacre Fellow of the Royal College of Physicians) regarding the approval of hospital posts suitable for general-practice training, which were milestones in our development. The formation of the General Practice Subcommittee of the Postgraduate Medical Education Council followed where, for the first time, the membership of this was divided equally between the General Medical Services Committee of the BMA and the College. This was later incorporated in the Joint Committee on Postgraduate Training for General Practice.

The management of the ever-lengthening Council agenda became a most pressing problem, until a 'starring' system was devised which allowed the agenda to be divided into items for information and those for debate.

The introduction of Denis Pereira Gray as Assistant Editor of our *Journal* was one of the many events during the first months of 1971. Later that year, 14 Princes Gate saw the visit of Senator Edward Kennedy, with his investigating team, researching for a health service for the United States of America.

The Senator had not been informed that he was to visit his former boyhood home when he called at the Royal College of General Practitioners. It was to be a surprise planned by his staff. This nearly led to a conflict with the security men, as the Senator insisted on jumping out of his official car (which was temporarily held up when turning into Princes Gate) when he recognized his former home. The Senator was somewhat bewildered at the red carpet and the official reception committee, but insisted on visiting a number of old haunts in the building, including the lift with its ancient mechanism. This visit lasted three and a half hours, including lunch.

The institution of the Sir Harry Jephcott General Practice Professorships, available for a period of several weeks to any British Medical School, was one of the ideas supported by Sir Max (later Lord) Rosenheim and funded by the Jephcott Trust and the Research Foundation of the College in conjunction with the prolonged leave regulations of the NHS. The impact of the Professorships at various medical schools was exceptional.

Co-operation with the other Royal Colleges was extended by the Obstetric Working Party with the Royal College of Obstetricians and Gynaecologists, the Report on *The General Practitioner in the Hospital* (jointly with the Royal College of Physicians), the appointment of a College member to a working party on Student Health at the Royal College of Physicians and the endowment of the Royal College of General Practitioners' Wolfson Travelling Professorship. All these indicated increasing trust in the academic capacity of the young College.

A meeting with Sir George Godber's team at the Department of Health and Social Security, regarding the selection and remuneration of teachers in general practice, was a further landmark. Much of what was later to be embodied in regulations and jointly agreed by the General Medical Services Committee of the British Medical Association and the Royal College of General Practitioners was outlined at that meeting.

The international spread of the College's influence and leadership in general-practice affairs was indicated by the Conference of North Sea Colleges during the 1971/72 Council year, initiated largely by the Northeast England faculty and the Dutch College of General Practitioners.

Some outstanding debates centred around the proposed abortion legislation, as well as on the evidence to the Robert Harvard Davis Committee set up by the Standing Medical Advisory Committee on Group Practice.

In March 1971 Lord Cohen of Birkenhead addressed our Council, as President of the General Medical Council, on the GMC's future and development, prior to the first Merrison Committee.

The event of the summer of 1972 was the launching of the book *Future General Practitioner: Learning and Teaching*[3]. One month later, 2500 copies had been sold. Subsequently a large number of reprints were ordered.

November 1 1972 marked the beginning of an exciting period for the College when much publicity was directed on it, and much evidence of its growing activities emerged. His Royal Highness The Prince Philip, Duke of Edinburgh, was installed on that day in the Hall of the Royal Geographical Society as an Honorary Fellow of our College and thereafter as President, an office which he held for one year. There was a large dinner at Grosvenor House, at which Prince Philip replied to the Toast of the College proposed by Lord Todd.

The College was kept in the news by a joint meeting with the Canadian College of Family Physicians in London later, and the scientific meeting and social activities connected with this, the presentation to John Hunt of the Victor Johnston Medal, the publication of the second edition of *General Practice Glossary*[4], the setting up of the Joint Committee on Contraception, the establishment of a John Hunt Fellowship and, finally, all our joy at John Hunt's ennoblement as Lord Hunt of Fawley. Later in the year, New Zealand Council was visited by Ian Watson as Deputy President and E. V. Kuenssberg as Chairman of Council, and helped towards independence as a sister College.

The problems of the European Economic Community also began to take up much of our time. Linguists and Europeans were at a premium in the British College, the few having to do much.

When the President, His Royal Highness The Prince Philip, Duke of Edinburgh, entertained to dinner the Presidents of the other Royal Colleges in the Damask Room at 14 Princes Gate, he led a debate on Continuing Education and Competence to Practice in the broadest interprofessional way.

John A. R. Lawson

Chairman of Council 1973

Patrick Byrne was elected President at the Twenty-first Annual General

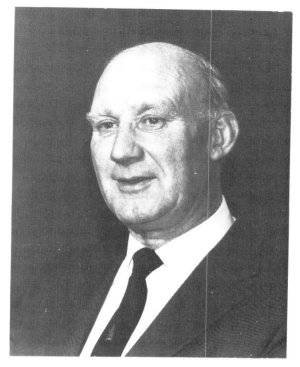

Plate 8   John A. R. Lawson 1973

Meeting on November 20 1973, and His Royal Highness The Prince Philip, Duke of Edinburgh, was installed as Patron, after his active year of office as President.

The years 1974–76 were years of consolidation within the College, when Council, regional councils, faculties, members and associates built on the work of previous years and considered the way ahead. In April 1974, the College held a five-day meeting to which representatives were invited from several European and North American countries to discuss problems connected with the measurement of quality in primary medical care. The conference, sponsored entirely by the Rockefeller Foundation, was held at the Foundation's villa in Bellagio, Italy. A paper on the proceedings was published in the College *Journal*[5].

Council debated a motion from the Midland Faculty on the inadequate consultation between Council and faculty boards. The importance of the work of the faculties to the College was fully endorsed. The faculty representative on Council was identified as the key person in this communication link between Council and the faculties, and he carried the

53

responsibility for the development and prosecution of College policy within the faculties. The honorary secretary of Council also arranged to hold regular meetings between faculty secretaries and himself at Princes Gate.

The interim report of the Oral Contraception Study[6] and the report of the Second National Morbidity Survey[7] were published during 1974.

A Postgraduate Committee of Council, chaired by the President, was set up in 1973 with the major task of approving those vocational training programmes and posts which furnished a learning experience suitable for assessment in the MRCGP examination. This committee later, at the request of the Chairmen of the Councils for Postgraduate Medical Education, formed the nucleus of the Joint Committee on Postgraduate Training for General Practice.

Council considered in detail the *Report of the Committee of Inquiry into the Regulation of the Medical Profession* (the Merrison Committee) and set up a working party to examine and report on that part dealing with the control of vocational training and the accreditation of individuals for general practice. The Report stated that,

General practice should be recognized as a specialty just like any other areas of medical practice.

The College strongly endorsed this view and Council agreed that recognition as a full specialty required general practice to accept new responsibilities for the standards of practitioners wishing to take part in training programmes.

During this period the College evidence to the Royal Commission on the National Health Service was prepared. This exercise gave us an opportunity to look at the present state and future needs of general practice. A number of members contributed by writing in with their own views and later commenting on the discussion document produced by Council.

Council was concerned with the somewhat tardy progress of the National Health Service (Vocational Training) Act. In company with the General Medical Services Committee of the BMA, the College was invited by the Department of Health and Social Security to a tripartite meeting to consider how the Act could be made to work with sense and flexibility.

The Court Report on *Child Health Services*, with its far-reaching implications for general practice, was published in 1976. Council debated the report in full and comments were sent to the Chief Medical Officer, Sir Henry Yellowlees.

In 1976, also, the opportunity was taken to purchase No 15 Princes Gate (see Chapter XV). The increased residential accommodation allowed many more members to stay at Princes Gate, and this was particularly welcome at a time when the cost of hotel rooms in London was rising fast.

Mention must be made of the deaths during this time of H. L. Glyn Hughes, CBE, DSO, MC (see Chapter XVI) and R. M. S. McConaghey, OBE. Glyn Hughes was Honorary Treasurer of Council for the twelve years following its foundation; Dr McConaghey was a member of the Foundation Council and founder editor of the *Journal of the Royal College of General Practitioners*. He remained as Editor until 1971.

Michael J. Linnett

Chairman of Council 1976

Michael Linnett took office at the beginning of the twenty-fifth year of the College. It was a time of pride in what had been achieved, but awareness that new tasks, generally perceived but yet to be defined, lay ahead.

During 1977 the Vocational Training Act was passed – a landmark in the evolution of postgraduate training for general practice. The accord achieved between the College, the General Medical Services Committee, the Joint Committee for Training in General Practice and the UK Conference of Regional Medical Advisers was remarkable.

A working party of Council convened by Donald Irvine produced written evidence for the Royal Commission on the National Health Service[8], and later gave oral evidence. The preparation of the documents involved a complete review of the role of general practice in health care, and of the College's own policy on standards and training; it proved to be a source paper in the debate on the College's future role which was initiated in the succeeding year.

The Education and Research Foundations were amalgamated in the new Scientific Foundation Board, under the chairmanship of Sir George Godber, with Sir Michael Swann and Professor Martin Vessey as extracollegiate members. The Board had assumed an important role in promoting and funding research projects.

Negotiations begun under John Lawson's chairmanship for the purchase of No 15 Princes Gate were successfully completed, and work began on the welding together of the two buildings to provide badly needed office space and further residential accommodation.

The Medical Recording Service, the brainchild of John and Valerie Graves, which was founded in 1958, had been so successful and its activities had become so widely spread throughout the medical professions that it was made a separate Charity. The new Graves' Medical Audiovisual Library became an institution in its own right, retaining close links with the College (see Chapter IX).

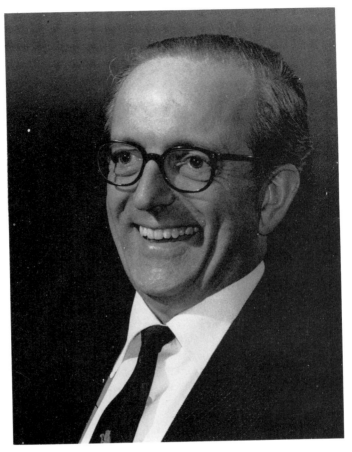

Plate 9   Michael J. Linnett 1976

The Twenty-fifth Annual General Meeting in 1977 was a special occasion. Kenneth Robinson, MP, remembered by many as an outstanding Minister of Health, was elected an Honorary Fellow, and the James Mackenzie Lecture was given by Denis Pereira Gray, the editor of the *Journal* of the College. His subject was 'Feeling at Home' – an appraisal of the value of home visiting in which he contrasted a current trend towards decline in home visits with the importance of the home in relation to health, and he warned that there was a danger of creating a vacuum in medical care. He said,

For me knowledge and understanding of the family, especially one with children, the elderly, the disabled, or the dying is always incomplete if I have never visited the home,

and he urged the continuation of home visiting as an integral part of general practice.

In his report on his year as chairman of the twenty-fifth Council of the College, Michael Linnett expressed the pleasure that he and the College felt that the honorary secretary of the Steering Committee, Foundation Council, and the first 13 College Councils had been his senior partner – John Hunt. The College's Silver Jubilee culminated its great achievement in establishing general practice as a medical discipline in its own right. It had marked the acceptance of educational methods and training for primary care. But it also pointed forward to a field of increasing importance, the evaluation of the care our patients receive, and the way in which general-practice knowledge and skills can be maintained and improved by continuing education and research. Thus the twenty-fifth year of the College ended with a debate on the College's role in the future.

References

1. MacLean, D. W. (1956). The influence of home conditions during the first five years of life on the physical and mental health of children. *Research Newsletter, NS* **3**, 47–62
2. Hunt, J. H. (1957). The Renaissance of General Practice. *Br. Med. J.,* **i**, 1075–1082
3. Royal College of General Practitioners (1972). *The Future General Practitioner. Learning and Teaching.* (London: British Medical Journal)
4. *Royal College of General Practitioners (1973). A general-practice glossary. J. R. Coll. Gen. Practit.,* **23**, Suppl. 3
5. Buck, C., Fry, J. and Irvine, D. H. (1974). A framework for good primary medical care – the measurement and achievement of quality. *J. R. Coll. Gen. Practit.,* **24**, 599–604
6. Royal College of General Practitioners (1974). *Oral Contraceptives and Health. An interim report from the Oral Contraception Study.* (Tunbridge Wells: Pitman Medical)
7. Royal College of General Practitioners, Office of Population Censuses and Surveys and Department of Health and Social Security (1974). *Morbidity Statistics from General Practice.* (London: HMSO)
8. Royal College of General Practitioners (1977). Evidence to the Royal Commission on the NHS. *J. R. Coll. Gen. Practit.,* **27**, 197–206

VI
REGIONAL FACULTIES AND REGIONAL COUNCILS IN THE UNITED KINGDOM

REGIONAL FACULTIES IN THE UNITED KINGDOM AND EIRE

Sylvia G. DeL. Chapman, John H. Hunt and Andrew Smith

From the start we were determined not to repeat the mistake, made more than a century ago, of excluding doctors outside London from College affairs and administration. We discussed this, and the possibility of having regional organizations of the College, several times before the Steering Committee met. F. M. Rose brought this matter up in the Steering Committee and the term 'regional faculties' was agreed. The important work of the regional faculties was described and discussed in detail in the first five *Annual Reports* of the College. At the end of each subsequent *Annual Report* a description of each faculty and of the work of its committees was given.

We believed that the College's regional organization would be of the greatest importance. Through it, not only would the College be able to assist nearly all its members and associates, wherever they might live and work, but would also be able to help the College, in return, by supplying information about their needs and about many other aspects of general practice with which the Council was concerned. Through the boards of the regional faculties it was hoped to develop a useful two-way channel for information and help. The Foundation Council was most anxious to ensure that every regional faculty would always be represented on the College Council.

59

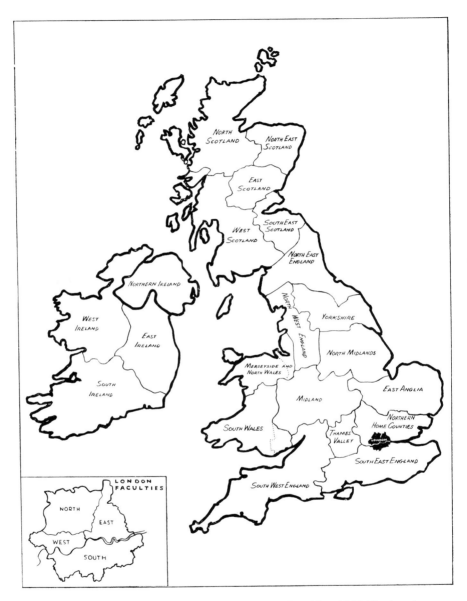

Plate 10 Approximate boundaries of the regional faculties, 1954. During the next 23 years several faculties changed their names or the areas they served

On March 28 and May 2 1953, statements were published in the *British Medical Journal*[1] and in *The Lancet*[2] on the proposed regional faculties of the College, and a map showed the distribution of members and associates at that time throughout the British Isles. For educational purposes, and to facilitate arrangements for postgraduate study and research, it was hoped that the headquarters of these regional faculties would be situated near the offices of the undergraduate or postgraduate deans or directors of local medical schools and of university research departments. In some places it was realized, however, that this might not be possible. It was felt that a close link with the universities would underline the academic nature of the College's work. There were, then, 16 universities with medical schools in England, Scotland, Wales and Northern Ireland – Aberdeen, Belfast, Birmingham, Bristol, Cambridge, Cardiff, Durham, Edinburgh, Glasgow, Leeds, Liverpool, London, Manchester, Oxford, Sheffield and St Andrews.

Pilot faculties were formed in the following places: Belfast, Birmingham, Bristol, Manchester, Newcastle-on-Tyne, with five in Scotland. It was agreed that the status of all regional faculties should be equal. In areas far away from a medical school or university, it was understood that subfaculties might be needed, as in Hull.

The list of proposed faculties in Great Britain and Eire and the areas served by them was drawn up, and can be seen on the map (Plate 10). Members and associates of the College were free to choose to which faculty they could most conveniently belong.

Duties of Faculties

The duties of faculties were to relieve the College Council of local responsibilities connected with activities of the College. These activities would deal largely with undergraduate education, postgraduate education and research, working in close liaison with the local medical school, and the postgraduate and research departments of the local university. It was expected that, later, many other functions of the College might devolve upon the faculties.

Boards of Faculties

The board of each faculty consisted of a chairman, deputy chairman, honorary treasurer and honorary secretary, and from seven to 22 other members, with up to five associates. Five was a quorum for meetings of the board. Each board could invite individuals from its local medical school, university or other relevant authority to assist in an advisory capacity.

61

Members of the board were elected annually by members of the faculty. Officers of the board were elected by the board itself. For special purposes, subcommittees could be elected by the board as and when required.

A Faculty Organisation Committee of Council was formed towards the end of 1953 with the following terms of reference:

> To supervise the establishment of faculties of the College in the United Kingdom and Overseas. To determine the boundaries of faculty regions and to recommend changes in these boundaries when desirable. To supervise the internal organisation of faculties and their relations with each other and with the Council of the College. To produce faculty registers of members and associates. To draw up the faculty constitution and confirm faculty byelaws; to consider any proposed alterations in these and to make recommendations to the Council thereon.

At the time of the First Annual General Meeting, on November 14 1953, ten pilot faculties had been established. By the end of June 1954 all 22 faculties in the British Isles had been founded. Each of these was represented on the Council of the College. As far as possible it was arranged that at least one member of the College Council was present at the inaugural meeting of each faculty. The Honorary Secretary of the College Council spoke at 12 of these inaugural meetings in England and Wales and at one in Ireland (Dublin), and the Vice-chairman of Council spoke at six of them.

It was decided that the head of each faculty should be called the Provost. Meetings of the board of a faculty were to be held at least quarterly.

The Committees of faculty boards were, at first, largely concerned with local arrangements for undergraduate education of medical students in the problems of general practice, with the organization of postgraduate lectures and courses for general practitioners (and in helping them to attend these courses) and with encouraging general-practitioner research. All this work was done in close liaison with the corresponding committees of the College Council and/or the local medical school. Each committee of a faculty board elected its own chairman and honorary secretary, and included in its membership perhaps four to six members and associates of the College, and a few non-members co-opted for special qualities from the local medical school, university or elsewhere.

Faculty bye-laws were drawn up. A conference of chairmen, honorary secretaries and honorary treasurers of faculties took place on October 19 1954.

The first faculty to be formed was the North-east England faculty

(April 4 1953), followed quickly by the Northern Ireland faculty (April 30 1953), the South-east Scotland faculty (May 3 1953), and the Midland faculty (May 13 1953). All the other Scottish faculties and the North-west England faculty were formed before the end of May 1953. It is interesting to note, now, that the first London faculties appeared in May and June 1954, more than a year after those mentioned above.

By September 30 1954, there were 22 faculties in the United Kingdom and two in Eire.

The enormous scope of the work done by the faculties is described in the annual reports – it included arranging lectures, semesters, discussions, local and county meetings, social meetings, student attachments to family doctors, with the continuing education of general practitioners by Sunday-morning ward rounds, refresher courses and other activities. Noted, also, was the great amount of help faculties gave to general practitioners in research (college-sponsored, faculty-sponsored and by individuals). Several faculties produced journals, gazettes, newsletters and news sheets.

By the end of 1967, when the College was 15 years old, there were 39 regional faculties – 24 at home and 15 overseas.

During its first quarter of a century the College had 46 faculties altogether at home and overseas. Some changed their names and some their boundaries to correspond with Regional Health Authorities. One, the Uganda faculty, had to drop out because of local problems. Thirteen changed over to the Australian and New Zealand Colleges, and to the South African Academy of Medicine. At the end of 25 years there were 30 home faculties and subfaculties. The names of officers and members of faculty boards and the chairmen of their committees and the work they have done are printed in the annual reports.

The development of overseas regional faculties and overseas regional councils is described in Chapter XXI.

REGIONAL COUNCILS IN THE UNITED KINGDOM AND EIRE

SCOTTISH COUNCIL

William S. Gardner, John M. Henderson and Richard Scott

At its meeting on March 8 1953, the Foundation Council of the College agreed to the formation of a Scottish Council

for the purpose of coordinating the regional faculties and other local organizations in Scotland, of maintaining liaison between the

Council of the College and these bodies and their members, of investigating matters peculiar to Scotland and of making recommendations thereon to the Council of the College.

Richard Scott of Edinburgh had been the only Scottish member of the Steering Committee of the College and therefore the initial spadework fell to him. He contacted Charles Fleming who was, at that time, a Senior Medical Officer at the Scottish Home and Health Department, with special responsibility for general practice. As such he knew, either personally or by repute, many of the principals in general practice in Scotland. Dr Fleming gave Richard Scott a list of doctors who, he felt, might be interested in establishing a Scottish Council of the College, and on May 15 1953 Richard Scott called a meeting of these doctors. At this meeting arrangements were made for the setting up of an interim Scottish Council.

Two Scottish members of the Foundation Council of the College chose from the five Health Service Regions in Scotland a foundation member of the College who was invited to arrange an inaugural meeting of a proposed faculty in each of these regions. A letter was sent to each foundation member and associate in Scotland telling of the plans made for the first meeting of a proposed faculty in his or her region. Such preliminary gatherings took place in each of the five faculty areas during the four weeks following the meeting in Edinburgh on May 15. At these meetings either Richard Scott or John Henderson attended to explain the purpose and workings of the College. As a result of the nominations received, a meeting was held in Edinburgh on June 11 1953, at which an interim Scottish Council of the College was formed with Richard Scott as honorary secretary and John Henderson as chairman. This Council consisted of two members from each of the South-east, East, North-east, and North Scotland regions and three members from the West of Scotland, in addition to the chairman, deputy chairman and honorary secretary of the Interim Scottish Council.

At this point it should be emphasized that the initiation, and for many years thereafter the smooth running, of Scottish Council was due primarily to the work of Richard Scott who was its Honorary Secretary from 1953 to 1969.

William Fulton of Glasgow did excellent work for the Scottish Council and for his faculty. He was responsible for much of the goodwill and co-operation between the College and the British Medical Association in Scotland.

The Interim Scottish Council decided that:

(1) Faculty boundaries should be the same as the boundaries of the National Health Service Regions. Many years later the Council of

the College adopted a similar plan when considering the re-organization of the College's faculty boundaries in England and Wales in the light of the 1974 National Health Service re-organization plans.

(2) Its chairmanship should rotate through the faculties.

Among many subjects discussed at meetings of the interim Scottish Council and its immediate successors was that of criteria for membership of the College, including the introduction of an examination. This subject is dealt with in detail in Chapter X. Suffice it to say that while all Scottish faculties were overwhelmingly in favour of the introduction of an examination at an early date (together with a substantial minority in Yorkshire and the Midlands holding the same opinion) the first College Council, having carefully considered the problem, was not in favour of introducing a membership examination at that stage.

It would be tedious to detail the many subjects dealt with by Scottish Council over the years. It was, and is, motivated by two guiding principles:

(1) To coordinate rather than to initiate the work in the faculties, receiving reports from them, helping with their projects when necessary and acting in liaison between faculty membership and the Council of the College in London.

(2) To produce evidence or comment on behalf of the College in Scotland on various aspects of medical policy when so asked by government departments or other organizations.

It was inevitable that, over a quarter of a century, events, some happy, some tinged with sadness, should have occurred in the life of Scottish Council.

In 1967 the Ian Dingwall Grant Award was started as a memorial to I. D. Grant of Glasgow, a well-loved figure in the West of Scotland, a member of Scottish Council since its earliest days, a prominent figure in BMA circles and the second President of our College. He died with tragic suddenness in BMA House in 1962. This award was made possible by the donation of a sum of money from the Caledonian Medical Society on the winding-up of its affairs. The interest on this donation makes possible a small award every other year to a young practitioner to 'extend his training experience by visits to other practices or institutions to help him to prepare for specific studies or investigations relevant to general practice'.

In 1972 the Allen and Margaret Wilson Lectureship was inaugurated. Allen Wilson was a valued member of Scottish Council who, with his wife Margaret, was tragically killed in a car accident in 1967.

In happier vein: (1) The badge of office for the Chairman of Scottish

Council, incorporating the Scottish Arms of the College, is a most attractive emblem. It was presented in 1970 by John Hunt as a personal gift symbolising 'his deep affection for his Scottish colleagues and in gratitude for all they have done for the College'. (2) In 1954 Scottish Council acquired a gavel, carved by Perthshire craftsmen from the wood of a tree which grew in the garden of the birthplace of Sir James Mackenzie. This gavel became known, unofficially, as 'The Hammer of the Scots'. Some years later, a stand for the gavel was presented by the North-east Scotland faculty. (3) On the occasion of the award by the university of Edinburgh of an Honorary Doctorate of Medicine to Dame Annis Gillie, a Past-President of our College, Scottish Council presented her and the College with a mace for College use on official occasions (see Chapter XIX). (4) A dinner was held in Edinburgh in 1978 to mark the silver jubilee of Scottish Council and the South-east Scotland faculty. At this dinner a gift of leather hand luggage was made to Richard Scott in appreciation of all his splendid work for Scottish Council as its honorary secretary from 1953 to 1969. (5) During the lifetime of Scottish Council the establishment of chairs of general practice in all four Scottish medical schools was completed, and a General Practice Unit was opened in Chalmers Hospital, Edinburgh. All four Scottish universities with medical schools sponsored official postgraduate courses, and the postgraduate education committees of faculty boards were active in helping to plan and run such courses.

The Scottish Home and Health Department gave a five-year grant to finance a general-practice research support unit at the University of Dundee.

The Coat of Arms of the College in Scotland

Extract of Matriculation of the Arms of The College of General Practitioners

WHEREAS a Petition on behalf of The Council of THE COLLEGE OF GENERAL PRACTITIONERS having been presented unto the Lord Lyon King of Arms of date 2nd February 1962 SHEWING: THAT, the said College of General Practitioners, is an unincorporated Association, formed on 19th November 1952, and has a Scottish Council for the co-ordination of the work of the said College in Scotland; THAT Letters Patent of date 20 June 1961 over the signatures of Garter, Clarenceux and Norroy and Ulster Kings of Arms granted certain Ensigns Armorial in favour of the said College of General Practitioners, together with Supporters granted by the said Garter; AND the Petitioners having prayed that the said Arms might now be matriculated in the Public Register of All Arms and Bearings in Scotland with such modification, if any, as might be requisite under the Laws of Arms in Scotland, the Lord Lyon King of Arms by Interlocutor of date 20th February, 1962 Granted Warrant to the Lyon Clerk to matriculate in the Public Register of All Arms and Bearings in Scotland in name of the said College of

General Practitioners the following Ensigns Amorial, videlicet: Per pale Sable and Argent, a chevron counterchanged between in chief an Opium Poppy Flower and a Gentian Flower, both slipped proper, and in base a Roman Lamp Orenflamed, also proper And on a wreath of these Liveries Argent and Sable is set for Crest an owl proper, supporting with the dexter claw a Gavel upright Or entwined with a serpent also proper, and on a Compartment below the Shield, along with this Motto "Cum Scientia Caritas" are set for Supporters, Dexter, a unicorn Or, armed, crined and unguled Argent: Sinister, a lynx proper, spotted Azure, Gules, Vert, Or and Argent, and Ducally gorged and chained of the last. Matriculated the 12th day of March 1962. Extracted fourth of the 43rd page of the 45th Volume of the Public Register of All Arms and Bearings in Scotland this 13th day of March 1962.

SIGNED AND SEALED
"H. A. B. LAWSON"
Lyon Clerk Keeper of the Records.

The main differences in the Scottish Council's Coat of Arms are: The owl is supported on a wreath of 'Liveries Argent and Sable' and not by a Helmet as in the English matriculated Coat of Arms; the Lynx on the left is 'spotted Azure, Gules, Vert, Or and Argent, and Ducally gorged and chained of the Last'. In other words the heraldic colouring of the Lynx is different and the position of the chain is different. The compartment below the shield with the opium poppy and gentian and Roman Lamp Orenflamed along with the motto "Cum Scientia Caritas" carrying the supporters is also of some slightly different shading and shape.

Chairmen of Scottish Council:

J. M. Henderson	1953	J. A. R. Lawson	1966
W. S. Gardner	1957	J. S. Scobbie	1969
Lowell Lamont	1960	R. Scott	1972
I. M. Scott	1963	D. E. Fraser	1975

WELSH COUNCIL

John H. Owen

The Welsh Council was founded on January 7 1968. The College had come to Wales through David Hughes of St Clears and Wilfred Howells of Swansea, both of whom were members of the Foundation Council of the College. Trevor Hughes carried the banner to North Wales, supported by E. Wynne Jones, but the nature of its geography, with a sparse and scattered population, made it necessary to annex North Wales to the Merseyside faculty.

On April 11 1954, John Hunt went to Cardiff to address a meeting of 33 Welsh members of the College, and as a result the Welsh faculty was formed.

The faculty included the counties of Glamorgan, Carmarthen, Cardigan, Pembroke, Brecon, Radnor, Montgomery and Monmouth. After some discussion with the Merseyside and North Wales faculty it was agreed that North Wales members in the counties of Anglesey, Caernarvonshire, Denbigh, Flint and Merioneth should be allowed to join whichever faculty they wished. Postgraduate facilities would be available in both North and South Wales.

One of the many highlights of this emerging faculty was a successful research symposium held in Cardiff under the chairmanship of Professor Harold Scarborough, then Professor of Medicine at the Welsh National School of Medicine. Several Geigy-sponsored symposia were organized in Wales. Pfizer-sponsored lectures were also eagerly awaited annual events. In the 1950s there were eminent lecturers such as Professor A. G. Watkins on 'Parents and Children', and E. Roland Williams from Pembroke on 'Physicians Extraordinary'. George Abercrombie visited in 1959 and lectured on 'The Perpetual Student', showing how a doctor learned first from his teachers and then during the whole of his professional life from his patients. Stephen Taylor (later Lord Taylor of Glyn Ceiriog) delivered a lecture entitled 'The Future of General Practice', and in 1964 the Pfizer lecture was given by David Zacharin, then Chairman of Council of the Australian College of General Practitioners. In 1970 E. V. Kuenssberg lectured on 'Practice Organization'.

The main event of the 1960s, however, was the 1967 Spring Meeting of the College held in Cardiff under the chairmanship of Lord Platt. This was the first meeting of the College as a 'Royal' College and a particular privilege to the Welsh faculty. The theme of the symposium was 'The early detection of endemic and imported disease'[3]. Annis Gillie, as President, insisted at the faculty dinner that the official Grace be translated into the native tongue. This was not surprising as her brother, Mr Blaise Gillie, had learnt the Welsh language during his term as the Senior Civil Servant in Wales. During the meeting the faculty was able to present to the College Appeal Fund a substantial sum of money collected mainly in covenants from its members.

Professor C. R. Lowe, from the Department of Social Medicine of the Welsh National School of Medicine, became a valuable supporter of the aims of the College, notably in research. W. O. Williams's enthusiasm in this field was infectious, and his study of 'Workload in South Wales' was but one of his many projects. His help and encouragement to aspiring general-practitioner research workers throughout Britain was well-known and appreciated. He continued to direct the College's research unit in Swansea.

Julian Tudor Hart's contributions over the years had been invaluable and his work became known internationally. Professor Peter Parish, during his stay in Swansea, contributed much to the understanding of the importance of research in general practice; and Dewi Rees's study of bereavement[4] and its associated problems was one of the first investigations of its kind.

Chiefly as a result of the influence and enthusiasm of John Parry, liaison with the Welsh National School of Medicine was established early, and several symposia were organized for medical students[5]. The theme of the first of these, on May 16 1962, was 'Anaemia'. Addresses were given by J. Fry, A. M. Revie and E. Scott[6].

During the early 1960s there were rumblings in the Welsh faculty that it had become too large, again for reasons of geography and topography, and difficulties were encountered in holding regular meetings of members from widely separated counties. The Welsh faculty representative of College Council at the time was John Owen. The Chairman of Council was Harry Levitt, whose encouragement was invaluable. In order to establish an all-Wales representation, attempts were made to form a separate North Wales faculty in addition to the South-east Wales faculty based on Cardiff, and a South-west Wales faculty based on Swansea. Enthusiasm for this was lacking in the North, where members felt more naturally aligned to Merseyside. Representation, however, was achieved by inviting the Chairman of the Merseyside and North Wales faculty and another representative to serve on Welsh Council. Padraig O'Brien was very proud of this Celtic connection and was the first to serve.

1973 was a notable year when Welsh Council held a symposium on 'The Community Hospital'[7] which was chaired by the then President of the College, HRH The Prince Philip, Duke of Edinburgh. His Royal Highness initially visited the General Practice Unit of the Welsh School of Medicine where he was shown both the service and educational activities of the Centre by the honorary director, Professor R. Harvard Davis, accompanied by Professor C. R. Lowe, an honorary fellow, and G. I. Watson, the Deputy President. His Royal Highness then took the chair for the morning session of the symposium at the University Hospital of Wales.

In 1974, Welsh Council held a combined meeting in Cardiff with the Welsh Division of the Royal College of Psychiatrists, under the chairmanship of Sir Martin Roth.

Following W. V. Howells in the Welsh Council chair were, in succession, David Coulter and John H. Owen. There had been three honorary secretaries of Welsh Council: D. J. Llewellyn, R. C. Humphreys (an active research enthusiast long before joining the College in 1956) and Derek Wilson.

The Welsh Council functions largely in a coordinating capacity for the faculties in Wales, but it had also itself promoted a number of projects, and established a fruitful liaison with Governmental and other bodies.

In the developing postgraduate area much work was done by David Coulter and Derek Llewellyn. The first vocational training scheme in Wales was based on Bridgend. Apart from establishing links with postgraduate centres through the Welsh faculties, a system of special interest groups was inaugurated, one of which thrived under the chairmanship of Margot Richards. Another important event was the publication in 1971 of a text-book of general practice specifically directed at vocational training, *The Practice of Family Medicine,* under the editorship of David Coulter and Derek Llewellyn, with 20 Welsh general practitioners contributing chapters[8].

The faculties inaugurated several prizes for written work – the South-west Wales faculty commemorated Donald Isaac with a prize for an essay on a chosen subject related to general practice; Bruce Lervy was the first winner, with an essay entitled 'Home visiting is essential to good general practice'[9]. The South-east Wales faculty instituted a prize for the under-graduate judged to have shown the most interest and ability in general practice in the final year of study at the Welsh National School of Medicine. The Welsh Council Prize was awarded annually for work by vocational trainees in general practice in the form of an essay or project report suitable for publication in the College *Journal.* Syntex Pharmaceuticals Ltd established four Fellowships in Rheumatology for trainers or the partners of trainers in Wales, called 'The RCGP Welsh Council/Syntex Fellowship in Rheumatology'.

The contribution of the Principality to family doctoring in general and to the College in particular will continue to grow and remain worthy of the industry and devotion of the College's past, present and future membership.

Chairmen of Welsh Council

J. N. M. Parry	
(chairman of Steering Committee)	1968
W. V. Howells	1968–71
D. F. Coulter	1971–74
J. H. Owen	1974–77

IRISH COUNCIL

James S. McCormick, John E. McKnight and Noel D. Wright

The Irish Council met for the first time on December 2 1962. Its first chairman was J. M. Hunter, vice-chairman G. C. Maguire and honorary secretary V. G. Doyle.

Irish Council had its beginnings in a request from College Council that the four Irish faculties appoint a Steering Committee 'to consider the establishment of an Irish Council of the College'. The Steering Committee first met in Belfast on April 30 1961. It met on three occasions and drafted a constitution which was subsequently approved by the Irish faculties and by the College Council.

The Irish Council was made up of three members from each faculty, elected by the faculties, with the addition of the Irish members of College Council. This gave a total membership of approximately 15.

Following the meeting in Cork it became the practice, still continuing, that the chairmanship should rotate between the faculties, each chairman serving for one year, continuity being provided by the honorary secretary and honorary treasurer each serving for a period of three years and being eligible for re-election. This arrangement provided for the development of a wide variety of educational and social activities.

The *raison d'être* for Irish Council was to provide a college focus for those matters concerning the College which were primarily peculiar to Ireland. While this applied with particular force to the faculties in the Republic who wished to make representation to Government, universities and other bodies, there were also issues in the North of Ireland which were, in a sense, domestic and not the concern of the College as a whole.

The most noteworthy result of the recognition was the creation in Northern Ireland of the Irish Institute of General Practice. This body was set up by the Council for Postgraduate Medical and Dental Education to accept responsibility for vocational and continuing education in general practice. It derived its membership mainly from the RCGP, the Irish Medical Association and the Medical Union. Almost predictably most of the members, regardless of which body they represented, were members or fellows of the College. The Institute may well become the recognized body of accreditation in general practice under the EEC Regulations.

It had become usual for Irish Council to be invited to comment on documents emanating from the Department of Health, and from time to time to give evidence. In short, Irish Council was recognized as the voice of the College in Ireland. Similarly, the Northern Ireland faculty was frequently consulted by Government and other bodies on general-practice matters and had become increasingly influential.

71

Another reason for establishing an Irish Council was that members in Ireland might more readily identify with the College. This was particularly important as, for many, Princes Gate was many miles away. This difficulty was reflected in the relatively large proportion of associates in the Republic. From time to time many people felt that an independent Irish College would be appropriate and it may be that this will happen in the future. Irish Council had to some extent diminished the pressure for independence, and in many people's eyes this was for the best.

One of the most important virtues of Irish Council was the partnership it entailed between Northern Ireland and the Republic. The regular cross-border traffic was a source of enormous enrichment and the unstinting help given to the faculties in the Republic by their colleagues in the North was extremely valuable.

During its lifetime Irish Council had the good fortune to welcome to its meetings many of the Presidents of the College. John Hunt attended its first meeting as honorary secretary of the College Council and subsequently as President. Dr Rose attended the Spring General Meeting in Dublin in 1964. On this occasion he and other members of Council were received by President De Valera. Annis Gillie visited Cork in 1966, G. I. Watson, Dublin in 1972, and P. S. Byrne, Galway in 1975.

A major event in the life of Irish Council was the acquisition of an address, secretarial assistance and suitable rooms for meetings at the Institute of Public Administration in Dublin. This arrangement, negotiated on favourable terms in 1971, continued.

Irish Council had been very fortunate in its officers, particularly in its chairmen.

Joe Hunter, the first chairman, was a remarkable man. A foundation member of the College, he epitomized all that was best in general practice. He had total integrity and enormous charity; he never said an unkind word. He had a lively and delicious sense of humour which was never malicious. Not a great talker in debate, his contribution always reflected concern and serious thought: not for him the cheap debating point. He guided the infant Council with great skill and continued to be a member until his death.

George Maguire, the second chairman, was cast in a very similar mould. Springing from a different tradition he embodied the same virtues and the same strengths. A great lover of the Irish language, he brought to Council a sense of a specific and valuable Irish contribution.

Ivor Hooper represented the urban rather than the rural aspects of practice. Self-effacing, peering through his glasses, he had an absolute sense of right and wrong. Although like some of his predecessors not a fluent debater, he shared with them a great sense of humour.

Stanley Boyd was the second chairman from the North. Quiet, unassuming and constant, he also embodied concern for his fellow men and women and the welfare of the College.

Irish Council has successfully represented the College in Ireland and has provided a focus for bringing together many doctors from all over the island. This was an enriching experience, not only in terms of formal educational exercises, but in the informal exchange of ideas and views, and in the cementing of friendship.

Chairmen of Irish Council

J. M. Hunter	1962–63	N. D. Wright	1970–71
G. C. Maguire	1963–64	A. F. Delany	1971–73
Ivor Hooper	1964–65	E. Waldron	1973–74
E. J. O'Brien	1965–66	J. F. Gowen	1974–75
A. S. Boyd	1966–67	G. T. C. Hamilton	1975–76
S. Flannery	1967–68	J. O. Mason	1976–77
V. G. Doyle	1968–69	P. D. O'Beirne	1977–78
O. K. Shorten	1969–70	M. O'Sullivan	1978–79

References

1. College of General Practitioners (1953). Regional Faculties. *Br. Med. J.,* i, 725
2. College of General Practitioners (1953). Foundation members of the College of General Practitioners. *Lancet,* ii, 894–895
3. Royal College of General Practitioners (1968). The early detection of imported and endemic disease. *J. R. Coll. Gen. Practit.,* 16, Suppl. 2
4. Rees, W. D. and Lutkins, S. G. (1967). Mortality of bereavement. *Br. Med. J.,* 4, 13–16
5. College of General Practitioners (1966). Mental illness in general practice. *J. Coll. Gen. Practit.,* 12, 233–238
6. College of General Practitioners (1963). Anaemia in general practice. *J. Coll. Gen. Practit.,* 6, 318–325
7. Royal College of General Practitioners (1973). The community hospital. *J. R. Coll. Gen. Practit.,* 23, 713–716
8. Coulter, D. F. and Llewellyn, D. J. (eds). (1971). *The Practice of Family Medicine.* (Edinburgh: E. & S. Livingstone)
9. Lervy, B. (1979). Home visiting is essential to good general practice. *South West Wales Faculty Annual Report*

VII
UNDERGRADUATE EDUCATION

James D. E. Knox and Andrew Smith

Some degree of training for the vocation of general practice had been taking place for a long time. Hippocrates taught it. In the last century doctors trained their assistants, and partners in general practice helped each other. Towards the end of the last century specialism was developing, but most specialists still did a certain amount of general practice and could teach this to their students. But as the specialties became more numerous and complex, teaching for general practice declined.

A certain amount of vocational training *was* taking place before and after the Second World War, apart from Geoffrey Barber and William Pickles lecturing about their work. At Charing Cross Hospital, when E. C. Warner was Dean, all students were encouraged to spend two weeks with a general practitioner, when possible in his home, during the course of their hospital training. Richard Scott's General Practice Teaching Unit in Edinburgh was just starting (1948) and others were thinking or working along similar lines for the future, but throughout the country special training for general practice diminished in all its stages – undergraduate, postgraduate and continuing education. It was no accident that William Pickles, Geoffrey Barber and Richard Scott played such prominent parts during the College's formative years.

Boundaries of faculties were drawn up to ensure that whenever possible there would be a medical school in the area of each, and in most instances faculty headquarters were situated close to a university. The interest that the College had in undergraduate affairs was expressed in the early days by the existence of an Undergraduate Education Committee of Council, and this structure was reflected at faculty level as well. This policy was later to prove its value, when medical schools were able to help to develop postgraduate education and, to a lesser extent, research.

The situation regarding undergraduate education, however, was rather different. Here was a field which had long been dominated by hospital medicine, in which liaison with general practice (with some notable exceptions) was far less developed. Whereas in postgraduate education and research in those days the College had received rather than given, in the field of undergraduate education it sought to offer service and assistance, but this it could not do unless invited. The newly formed Undergraduate Education Committee of Council, under the chairmanship of Geoffrey Barber, therefore set about finding ways to stimulate activity at faculty level[1].

An important document was published in 1953[1], setting out the case for educating undergraduates in those aspects of general practice best taught by general practitioners. The document examined arrangements existing at that time for such teaching in the medical schools in the United Kingdom. This makes a fascinating contrast with the bulky Gazetteer of Departments of General Practice published some 28 years later[2]. The first report discussed ways of encouraging further liaison between medical schools and general practitioners, and put forward the following recommendations:

(1) All medical students should be given an insight into general practice by general practitioners.
(2) Medical schools should co-opt general practitioners to advise and take part in the teaching of students.
(3) General practitioners who wished to co-operate should notify the dean of the medical school or the College of General Practitioners.

This last recommendation enabled the College to produce a register of those interested in undergraduate teaching. By 1958 it contained the names of more than 1300 volunteers: more than 450 of these general practitioners were willing to have students remain in their practices for a period of a week or more, while the remainder were willing to take students from the nearest medical school on a day-to-day basis on a number of occasions each year. The register was broken down on a regional basis, and local lists giving full particulars were available to faculties and others.

The Undergraduate Education Committee then set itself the task of surveying the medical curriculum in the light of the professional experience of members of the College (1954)[3], with the following conclusions:

(1) The last two years of school (secondary education) should be divided between receiving a broad education and an introduction to the scientific method.

(2) The present method of selecting medical students could be improved by co-opting a general practitioner on to each selection board.

(3) The medical curriculum requires revision so as to give students a broader introduction to all branches of medicine, including general practice.

(4) The present division between pre-clinical and clinical subjects is too sharp.

(5) There is a tendency for too much time to be spent at present on obscure subjects and highly technical procedures to the exclusion of a study of common disorders.

(6) Medical students should be given more insight into medicine as it is practised *outside* hospitals.

Much of this thinking was reflected in the *Report of the Royal Commission on Medical Education* (the Todd Report) (1968)[4]. The policy of the General Medical Council is to leave each medical school as free as possible to develop its own curriculum. The young College believed that the most effective way of influencing undergraduate education was to encourage local faculties to foster links with medical schools while, centrally, the College remained willing to respond to any requests from a medical school. It was deemed inappropriate at that stage to initiate action from head-quarters. This policy was to pay off eventually, though a decade was to pass before the College's advice was sought in the setting-up and the filling of Chairs of General Practice in the medical schools. Later still the College was invited to nominate a representative to the Court of at least one university.

Encouraged by the response of its membership to issues of under-graduate education, Council submitted to the General Medical Council in 1955 a list of 11 different recommendations based on the two earlier reports. Included in the document was a recommendation that a Department of General Practice be set up in each medical school. Possible roles and functions of such a department were succinctly outlined and are valid reading 25 years later. Anxious to maintain the momentum, the Undergraduate Education Committee, by now under the chairmanship of Richard Scott, brought together the three documents referred to above in a booklet entitled *On Undergraduate Education and the General Practitioner* (1958)[5]. A copy of this document was sent to the dean of each medical school in the United Kingdom and Eire.

ACADEMIC GENERAL PRACTICE

During the 1950s the foundations were being laid of the developing academic discipline of general practice. Among several prominent college members, Richard Scott made an outstanding contribution in presenting general practice not merely as a conglomeration of parts (some might have said the simpler parts) of other disciplines. He showed that teaching general practice involved an approach to clinical medicine which focuses attention on *the patient* rather than on the disease; that it involves *routine health care* as well as crisis treatment. General practice deals with patients in 'open society' in contrast to the more controlled environment of hospital[6] (1978).

Such moves helped to define areas in which contributions could be made from general practice, and to fit such potential teaching into the existing structure of undergraduate medical training. In doing so, the College was to play a vital part in contributing to what may be the most important single development in medical education since the Flexner Reports – namely a change of direction of undergraduate education, from producing at graduation a safe type of doctor (the 'utility' model) to producing a doctor still to be trained further (the 'basic' model) in whichever discipline career choice might lie, including general practice. This change of emphasis expressed in the Todd Report (1968) of course owed much to the development of a strongly positive College policy towards what has come to be known as 'vocational training'. The provision of educational objectives for such postgraduate training provided something positive to place alongside the longer-established, mainly hospital-based, specialties. Ten years earlier, however, the College had stated its view that 'the primary duty of medical schools is not to turn out ready-made general practitioners or specialists'.

The 1960s

Having formulated these ideas, the College now sought to promote their wider acceptance. By 1960 other major educational issues had presented themselves for consideration. The most urgent of these was vocational training for general practice. To enable the College to deal more effectively with these matters, Council absorbed its Undergraduate Education Committee into an Education Committee of Council, and faculty structure followed suit.

Building on the foundations laid in the 1950s, the College was enabled to make significant contributions to a number of key documents which were to have considerable impact on both the provision of health services and medical education. The first of these publications was the report entitled

The Field of Work of the Family Doctor (the Gillie Report of 1963)[7], published by the Standing Medical Advisory Committee of the Central Health Services Committee, the chairman of which was later to become President of the College – Dame Annis Gillie.

This document was to pave the way for the 'new charter' for general practice. The resulting changes in the terms and conditions of service of general practitioners working in the National Health Service did much to raise further the standard of care of patients. The Gillie Report did more than this – it brought before the profession and the public in a condensed yet readable form the very substance of general practice. A basis from which academic general practice could develop was now made more explicit. The views expressed owed much to research which had, in many instances, been initiated by and carried out by the College. In addition, the report contained a splendid summary of the relationship which ought to exist between general practice and the various other parts of the educational spectrum. The way was thus paved for the introduction of such developments as paid study leave for principals in NHS general practice.

Another document of major importance in the 1960s was the *Report of the Royal Commission on Medical Education* (1968). The College published separately, in 1966[8], the evidence which it submitted to the Royal Commission. Much of this was concerned with developing and implementing ideas on vocational training.

The 1970s

Early in 1970 the Education Committee of Council published the first clear statement on educational objectives of undergraduate teaching in general practice. Such objectives were included under two headings as follows:

(1) *Clinical aims*

   (a) To widen the student's understanding of patterns of disease.

   (b) To demonstrate problem definition and patient management, taking into account physical, psychological and social elements in the situation.

   (c) To illustrate aspects of care of patients with chronic disease.

   (d) To show the contribution that the general practitioner makes to the prevention of disease, promotion of health and early diagnosis.

   (e) To deepen the student's understanding of the doctor/patient relationship in general practice.

(2) *Professional aims*

    (a) To enable the student to understand general practice and its ways of working as a professional discipline.

    (b) To afford the student opportunities in the presence of general-practitioner teachers to develop an informed critical approach to the service provided for patients.

    (c) To assist medical schools in their attempts to promote a holistic approach to medicine.

PROFESSORIAL APPOINTMENTS

By now, medical schools both in the United Kingdom and throughout the Western world were beginning to respond to the ideas of the College. Edinburgh had already instituted its own fully autonomous Department of General Practice, with Professor Richard Scott as the first incumbent of the Sir James Mackenzie Chair of Medicine in relation to General Practice in 1963. Shortly thereafter Ian McWhinney, a family doctor from Stratford-upon-Avon, went to Canada as first holder of the Chair of Family Practice in the medical school of the University of Western Ontario at London, Ontario.

    It was not until the 1970s, however, that the movement spread more widely to United Kingdom medical schools – Dundee in 1970, then Manchester, Queen's University, Belfast and Sheffield in 1972 – soon to be followed by many others. All these senior academic appointments were filled by College members and fellows (for by now the fellowship had come into being). It is also probable that the increasing respect which the College now commanded (with the right to the prefix 'Royal') carried weight with university appointing committees, to which in most instances the Royal College was being invited to send representatives.

THE SIR HARRY JEPHCOTT PROFESSORSHIP

Awareness by the College of the change of heart being exhibited by the medical schools led E. V. Kuenssberg (then honorary secretary to the Research Foundation Board) in 1972 to formulate ideas on how this new situation could be further developed. He found a ready and generous supporter in the late Sir Harry Jephcott, who donated a sum of money for the express purpose of enabling distinguished family doctors to contribute their special skills and experience in the everyday life of selected universities for a limited period. Universities in the United Kingdom were invited to apply, and arrangements for the appointment were worked out jointly. This innovation owed part of its success to the generous provision for study leave open to principals in NHS general practice, a scheme which in turn was a by-product of the new Charter to which reference has already been made.

The first holder of the new Visiting Professorship to Glasgow was Keith Hodgkin of Redcar (later to be appointed first Professor of Family Practice in the Memorial University of Newfoundland).

One of the aims of the Sir Harry Jephcott Professorship was to encourage universities to develop the contribution from general practice to the medical schools' teaching. It is probably no coincidence that, shortly after Professor Hodgkin's period at Glasgow, a decision was taken to institute a fully autonomous Department of General Practice with a professor as Head at that medical school.

THE PUBLIC WELFARE FOUNDATION

Early in 1957 the Public Welfare Foundation of America made a donation of £320 to help promote the aims of the College in respect of undergraduate education. Council used this money to institute a competition among senior medical students in the United Kingdom and Eire (a further allotment of prize money was set for a similar development in Australia and New Zealand). Thus was born *The College's Undergraduate Essay Competition*. The conditions have been modified in recent years to allow a greater latitude to students, who need not now be in their final clinical years. Response to this competition has been consistently good, and some excellent studies have been produced.

Over the years the faculties have fostered relations directly with students in their local medical schools by a variety of activities, including social gatherings and joint educational endeavours, such as symposia relating to general practice. One feature of the 1970s was a growing interest by students and medical schools in career opportunities. In many instances students themselves undertook to organize 'careers fairs' at which different disciplines, now including general practice, contributed exhibits setting out career prospects.

In 1974, thanks to the generosity of the Cardew-Stanning Foundation, a mobile exhibit on career prospects in general practice was produced. This toured the country and formed a focus for College members in faculty areas to meet medical students and to engage their interest. For many years the College has assisted medical students wishing, on their own initiatives, to find an attachment to a general practitioner interested in teaching.

THE FUTURE

At the present time nearly all medical students in Great Britain have an opportunity of experiencing at first hand some of these educational contributions possible from the growing discipline of general practice. In 1977, in this country, there were 16 Professors of General Practice, and there was an extensive and increasing flow of literature relating to the undergraduate scene. With many of the College's goals then achieved, was there still a role for the College in the undergraduate educational scene? The answer was surely 'yes', as illustrated by Professor Patrick Byrne's excellent example in his teaching practice department in Manchester, and also work being done by many others. The following is a personal expression of opinion concerning ways in which the College continue to be involved.

(1) At the simplest level, by continuing to foster among general practitioners a spirit of enquiry, the College would assist medical schools by ensuring a network of educationally aware general practitioners, from whose ranks will come the tutors of the future.

(2) The College could give advice on broader educational issues, such as the changing relationship between vocational training and undergraduate education in a way that would not be possible otherwise.

(3) The College could continue to act as a catalyst for bodies such as the General Medical Council and possibly the University Grants Committee. By providing up-to-date information from everyday general practice, viewed from an educational and research standpoint, the College could assist these institutions in their ongoing tasks in re-adapting educational policy.

(4) Because of its early lead in developing academic general practice, the College was in a position to continue to assist other countries by contributing from experience gained in all medical education. An example of such a contribution can be seen in the work of the group of university teachers from eleven European countries – the Leeuwenhorst Group. This group published a series of documents, one of which presented an agreed summary of possible contributions which general practice might make to undergraduate education in medical schools in Europe[9].

(5) By complementing and supplementing university-based research with work arising from its own membership, the College could help to ensure that developing university departments of general practice were in a position to play their parts in teaching research

methods, while remaining in touch with practical issues of day-to-day care of patients, and did not become 'ivory towers'.

References

1. College of General Practitioners (1953). The teaching of general practice by general practitioners. *Br. Med. J.,* **ii,** 36–38
2. Murdoch, J. C. (ed). (1981). *A Gazetteer of Departments of General Practice in the British Isles.* 3rd edn. (Dundee: Association of University Teachers of General Practice)
3. College of General Practitioners (1954). Medical curriculum. Report of the Undergraduate Education Committee of the First Council. *Br. Med. J.,* **i,** 1146–1149
4. Todd Report (1968). *Royal Commission on Medical Education 1965–68. Report.* (London: HMSO)
5. Scott, R. (1958). Undergraduate education and the general practitioner. *Br. Med. J.,* **ii,** 577–580
6. Hodgkin, K. (1978). *Towards Earlier Diagnosis in Primary Care.* 4th edn. (Edinburgh: Churchill Livingstone)
7. Gillie Report (1963). *The Field of Work of the Family Doctor.* (London: HMSO)
8. College of General Practitioners (1966). *Evidence of the College to the Royal Commission on Medical Education.* Reports from General Practice 5. (London: CGP)
9. European Conference on the Teaching of General Practice (1978). The contribution of the general practitioner to undergraduate medical education. *J. R. Coll. Gen. Practit.,* **28,** 244–252

VIII
POSTGRADUATE EDUCATION AND VOCATIONAL TRAINING

PART I: 1953–1965

George Swift

'It was once true that the practice of medicine did not greatly change between qualification and retirement; but nothing could be further from the truth now.' Awareness of the accuracy of this quotation from the *Report of the Steering Committee* was probably the most important reason why so many doctors became Foundation Members of the College.

BEGINNINGS

In 1952 the impact of the pharmacological revolution, of sophisticated surgery of the heart and lung, and the dawning understanding of the relationship between the emotions of a patient and his symptoms, were stimulating general practitioners to search for ways in which they could learn about this new knowledge from experts, and discuss it with their colleagues. At this time there were no postgraduate centres or libraries in general hospitals open to practitioners. A few very large towns had medical institutes; in other places there was a medical society which had monthly meetings in the winter months, and many BMA Divisions would arrange occasional lectures. Courses under Section 63 of the NHS Act were beginning to be arranged by the British Postgraduate Medical Federation of the University of London and by some of the provincial medical schools. In a few places small groups of general practitioners were meeting together to discuss clinical problems, and one or two had developed into more formal societies.

It was clear that one of the main tasks of the new College was to attempt to define the needs for continuing education and, having defined them, to decide how best they could be achieved. It was significant that the committee charged with this task by the Foundation Council, under the chairmanship of James Simpson of Cambridge, was named 'The Postgraduate Education and Regional Organisation Committee'. The College centrally could collect evidence, act as a forum for discussion and exchange of ideas and provide general stimulation, but the provision of opportunities would rest upon the faculties working in close co-operation with their local medical schools, with the BMA and with other authorities.

The major needs defined by the Foundation Council were:

(1) In training a qualified doctor for a career in general practice.
(2) In continuing a practitioner's education throughout his career.
(3) In encouraging general practitioners to follow a special bent.
(4) In providing a centre where general practitioners could meet.

Over the years, with the possible exception of the third, these objectives have largely been met. The College provided much of the necessary stimulation, though much of the executive role is now undertaken by postgraduate centres and the regional postgraduate committees.

THE FIRST POSTGRADUATE EDUCATION COMMITTEE

In 1954 The First College Council separated postgraduate education from faculty organization. Under Annis Gillie, the postgraduate education committee continued to study fundamental needs. The first task was to find out what arrangements were already made for postgraduate education throughout the country. In this, the committee was helped by the postgraduate committees of the faculties and acknowledgement is made in the Annual Report to the help given by the Director of the British Postgraduate Medical Federation of the University of London – Sir Francis Fraser. It became apparent that, though the postgraduate deans throughout the country were arranging a considerable number of courses, 'programmes of lectures and demonstrations tend to be too little linked to the realities of general practice, especially to that part of a family doctor's work which must be carried out in patients' homes' (1954 College *Annual Report*).

Many faculty committees were by this time changing the content of courses by influencing the organizers; some postgraduate deans had agreed to become co-opted members of committees and, in turn, representatives of faculties were in some cases co-opted to the Universities' Regional Post-graduate committees. The College and its faculties were now influencing the quality and quantity of postgraduate education.

Responsibility to Young Doctors

The committee also began to consider its responsibility to young doctors about to enter, or recently entered, into general practice – particularly young associate members. It suggested short introductory courses for possible entrants, courses to supplement the 'trainee system' and support for young single-handed principals. Finance and the lack of suitable premises delayed the possibility of putting some of these ideas into practice. Much thought was given to the idea of establishing an Institute of General Practice; and very tentative discussions took place on linking this with the West London Hospital on the site of a disused railway yard in Chelsea which later might include other medical institutes. Apart from courses for young and established doctors, such an institute would train secretaries and technical assistants and would study practice premises, organization and equipment. It was agreed that an Equipment and Premises Committee of Council should be set up.

No institute, however, appeared, but the fundamental principles of Annis Gillie and her committee have, over the years, been established in other ways: by the development of University Departments of General Practice; the establishment of Postgraduate Centres; the development of vocational training through the work and researches of many individuals in the faculties and the research organization of the College.

Questionnaire on Continuing Education

The Third Annual Report (1955) of the committee was little more than two pages in length. An extensive questionnaire on continuing education was prepared and circulated to all members and associates, the results of which were published on the authority of the committee in the *Journal* of the College during 1957–58[1].

Symposia

The first symposium, at the time of the annual general meeting, was organized by the committee for Sunday, November 20 1955. The subject, for the morning, was the scope and experience of the general-practitioner obstetrician which was causing major concern to the committee and many of the faculties. Twenty-five years later there have been great changes in the practice of obstetrics, but concern for the role of the general practitioner in this branch of medicine is no less.

In the afternoon the conference discussed 'The Practical Aspects of Postgraduate Medical Education in the Faculties'. No fewer than six deans and postgraduate deans attended as guest speakers. The morning session was published as a supplement to *Research Newsletter No 10*[2] and the afternoon session in *No 12*[3].

Gathering Data

During this year Harry Levitt, subsequently a chairman of Council, joined the committee as registrar and began the mammoth task of collecting information from the faculties on all postgraduate activities and dispersing this information as a source of ideas throughout the College. From this developed the *Monthly Postgraduate Information Diary* for the metropolitan regions.

The Fourth *Annual Report* (1958) starts with a section on educational activities in the faculties. For this the Council's Postgraduate Committee took no credit except that the faculties may have been stimulated by encouragement from Council. The number of new ventures was impressive, and it was clear that many faculties were now gaining the support of postgraduate deans and were able to influence the ways in which Section 63 finance was used.

Most of the 1956 Annual Report was concerned with the results of the educational questionnaire, to which more than 2000 answers had been received. Section IV of the questionnaire was concerned with the role of the general practitioner in obstetrics, and the evidence here was of immediate value. The Ministry of Health had set up a committee of inquiry into the maternity services of England and Wales (which produced the Cranbrook Report)[4] and had invited the College to give evidence. Council asked its Postgraduate Committee to prepare evidence, and this was based on the symposium in November 1955 and Section IV of the questionnaire. This was the first time the Postgraduate Committee had prepared evidence for an official enquiry and, so far as the writer can remember, the first report to an official body made by the College. The evidence was published in *Research Newsletter No 13*[5] (November 1956) and with minor modifications reads much as a report from the College in the 1980s might read. Whether this shows that the College has been successful is debatable, but it does suggest that the early Councils had foresight for present-day problems.

The educational questionnaire covered a much wider field than continuing education and training for practice. Much was discovered about what was being done by general practitioners at that time; how many had hospital appointments or worked part-time for industry; what access they had to pathology and X-ray diagnosis; how much help they had from nurses and secretaries; if they had experience of teaching or lecturing, and whether they would be willing to help run courses were amongst the subjects covered. The results were published in *Research Newsletter No 15–No 20*[1] in a series of papers by Robert Harkness and John and Valerie Graves.

Of particular value was the section dealing with the trainee scheme, with which over half of those answering were dissatisfied. The selection and training of teachers, the nature of training and the possibility of exploiting trainees were giving rise to great anxiety. There was a strong belief that training should be controlled by an educational rather than a service body. The evidence was of great help to the College when it began, later, a serious study of vocational training. Twenty-two years later many of the problems were still with us, but much had been learnt and achieved over the years.

Continuing Education and Faculties

The evidence in the answers to the questionnaire was of value to John Hunt and members of the postgraduate committee in preparing a document, *The Continuing Education of General Practitioners and the Work of a Postgraduate Education Committee of a Faculty Board*. This document was debated by officers of faculty Postgraduate Committees at a conference in July 1956.

Much of the document is as relevant today as it was then:

Contents of courses.

Over the years all subjects of importance to family doctors should be reviewed in these courses. The practical aspects of these subjects in relation to the work of family doctors should be emphasized, especially those connected with new methods of diagnosis and treatment. Social medicine, preventive medicine, industrial medicine, occupational diseases and rehabilitation must not be omitted.

Special needs.

It must be clearly understood that these special courses need to be different and distinct from those for consultants, because they should be strictly confined to those aspects of the special subject which a family doctor, still in active general practice, sees; details of highly-technical procedures, of interest and importance to consultants, may be largely omitted.

The educational value of working in a general practice.
General practitioners should carry on their general practices as efficiently as possible. There are few better methods of continuing the education of family doctors than for them to be working in a good partnership or group practice, or in a general-practitioner hospital meeting their colleagues, and discussing their difficult cases, as often as possible.

The role of Faculty Boards and their Committees.
It is not intended to make the College a 'closed shop'; other practitioners may, whenever possible, be invited to attend faculty-sponsored postgraduate activities. A faculty board's first responsibility is to its members and associates, but it must be remembered that one of the best ways of increasing the prestige of the College will be to render widespread services.

Annis Gillie's distinguished service as chairman of the Postgraduate Committee ended in 1956 when she became Vice-chairman of Council. Under her leadership the committee had established the principles, aims and needs of continuing education and vocational training which are still held by the College. She was succeeded by George Swift.

Help from others

In 1957 the College first began to receive major support from the pharmaceutical industry, much of this being related to postgraduate education. The Pfizer Grant provided £30 a year for each faculty (a considerable sum in those days), which was used to finance symposia and open lectures by distinguished speakers. This grant allowed faculties to develop independently in their own ways, and it was continued annually until recently, by which time it had become customary for faculty symposia to be financed by postgraduate deans – provided that the meetings were open to all doctors.
The Upjohn Travelling Fellowships also started in 1957. Originally these grants of up to £200 were limited to members of the College for any postgraduate education which could not be paid for with Ministry of Health grants; prolonged study leave and individual grants under Section 63 did not then exist. At that time it was calculated that £200 would provide course fees, travel and expenses for two weeks in a first-class hotel for the applicant and his wife. The postgraduate committee was responsible for

selecting the successful applicants for these awards and it soon became apparent that they could best be used to learn something that would enable the holder to carry out an investigation or research which would be of value to general practice as a whole. The awards are still made annually and it is fascinating to read the names of early holders who have subsequently come to the fore in College Council and the faculties and in departments of general practice. Often their special abilities relate directly to their Upjohn Awards.

In 1957 John and Valerie Graves approached the College with original ideas for recording lectures on gramophone records, as discs were known at that time, or on newly emerging tapes (see Chapter IX).

By chance Robin Pinsent met an old Cambridge friend who was working with Smith, Kline and French Ltd, and looking for a project to help the College. This friend was introduced to the chairman of the Postgraduate Committee who recognized him as a friend from a small Worcestershire village where they had both grown up. Thus was born the *Medical Recording Service* of the College, which was a responsibility of the Postgraduate Committee until an independent foundation was established (Chapter IX).

The fourth venture with which the Postgraduate Committee was involved was the Geigy Symposia. Following a symposium on Obstetrics attended by 600 doctors organized by the Northwest England faculty and financed by Geigy Ltd, the company offered to finance three such symposia annually – the Postgraduate Committee to select the faculty and approve the subject. These three symposia went on for many years. The first was held at Torquay in May 1961 on 'Emotional Disease in General Practice'[6]. That held by the East of Ireland Faculty in Dublin in 1964 established the tradition of a Spring General Meeting of the College.

There had always been considerable overlap of the educational plans of the four London, the Northern Home Counties and South-east England faculties, for all of which the British Postgraduate Medical Federation (BPMF) of the University of London was the University Postgraduate Authority. In 1957 the Postgraduate Joint Advisory Committee was formed to advise on and coordinate activities of the Metropolitan area. That committee continued until 1964 and was chaired first by Harry Levitt and later by Alec Bookless. Its main achievement was to develop relationships with the British Postgraduate Medical Federation on which the Committee was represented by Brigadier Donald Bowie and later also by A. A. G. Lewis, both regional advisers. A tradition was started of organizing a large number of 'refresher' courses in the week before the Annual General Meeting of the College. Donald Bowie was particularly helpful in arranging the earliest courses for trainers and young entrants to general practice. As mutual confidence grew, the BPMF began to recognize the College as an official organizer of courses. From it, the Headquarters Courses Sub-committee eventually emerged. The Joint Committee also arranged evening clinical meetings at the College when it moved to Princes Gate, but these were never well supported. When postgraduate centres began to be established, Alec Bookless, on behalf of the Postgraduate Committee, constructed the first national register of centres with the help of the honorary secretaries of faculties.

TRAINING FOR GENERAL PRACTICE

During 1958 the committee for the first time began seriously to study some of the problems of training for general practice. In the annual report it noted that many clinical conditions are not seen in hosptial and that the management of patients in general practice is often different from that in hospital. With the help of Alan Laidlaw the committee produced a booklet, *Memorandum for the Guidance of Trainers*[7]. I believe this was the first publication suggesting that there was any need for the teachers to be taught. We did not, because we could not, give any guidance; but we did try to indicate areas of practice management and of the services which could help patients which should be discussed with trainees – subjects which later became more formalized in area 4 (Medicine and Society) and area 5 (The Practice) in the publication *The Future General Practitioner* (1972).

1959 was a year of routine consolidation, but it is of interest to note that mention is made in the report of experiments in vocational training being carried out in Inverness and Wessex. The Committee made more contribution than it realized to these schemes, particularly in Wessex where I was able to implement some ideas which the Committee had discussed informally. The Postgraduate Joint Advisory Committee proved its worth when it organized with the BPMF, in May 1960, a conference on 'Teaching Methods in Formal Courses for the Continuing Education of Family Doctors'. This was the first conference where it was recognized that the content of lectures for general practitioners needed to be somewhat differ-ent from lectures to undergraduates or specialists. All the consultants who were organizing courses in the Metropolitan Regions were invited, and seven of the eight subjects were introduced by general practitioners.

Another Questionnaire

Following a previous questionnaire of 1956, a further questionnaire on postgraduate education was circulated with the College *Journal* in 1960. The purpose was to examine the adequacy of opportunities for study and to find out what the members and associates were really doing. The results of about a thousand replies were published in an article by John and Valerie Graves in the College *Journal* in May 1961[8]. The situation seemed to have improved since the previous questionnaire. The content of courses was more relevant to general practice. The most popular subjects remained the same and many of the courses were overbooked. Difficulties in getting away from the practice, and the problems of travelling to meetings, were common complaints. Practitioners were disagreeing with the belief of many organizers that the number of those attending was a measure of the success of a course. The demand for smaller meetings in which those attending could participate was increasing. At that time most courses took place in the major teaching centres and the answers to the questionnaire reflected the need for educational opportunities in all general hospitals. This was to be met before long by the establishment of postgraduate centres.

Although specific questions about meeting the criteria for continuing membership of the College had not been asked, it appeared that about 10% of members and 20% of associates had not fulfilled them and there was doubt about a further 20% of members and associates. It is interesting to reflect on what might have happened had Council chosen to enforce the criteria for continuing membership.

In 1961 it was becoming increasingly apparent that there were areas of common interest to the Undergraduate and Postgraduate Committees and a combined meeting was held. From this emerged the ideas which later resulted in the setting up of an Education Committee of Council responsible for all stages of education.

The Christ Church Conference

The College was invited to send a representative to the conference on postgraduate education organized by the Nuffield Provincial Hospitals Trust at Christ Church, Oxford, in December 1961. The Royal Colleges were represented by their Presidents but the College of General Practitioners sent the chairman of the Postgraduate Committee. John Fry, a trustee of the Nuffield Provincial Hospitals Trust, and I were the only general practitioners present. However, key roles were played by Gordon McLachlan, Donald Bowie, John Revans (later Sir John) and Sir George Godber, all of whom became later Honorary Fellows of the College.

Following the conference the Trust supported the movement to establish postgraduate centres in all general hospitals. This was probably the single most important step in developing vocational training and continuing education for general practitioners.

In June 1962, the Postgraduate Committee of Council followed up the Christ Church conference by a meeting of faculty representatives. The meeting was also attended by representatives of the Ministry of Health, Department of Health for Scotland and British Postgraduate Medical Federation, and representative deans of medical schools. Useful discussions took place on the possible and necessary developments in training for practice, and continuing education. Opening College speakers included Kenneth Foster, Bill Hylton, George Little and Valerie Graves.

Using Princes Gate

By 1963 the College was established at 14 Princes Gate and it was natural that the Postgraduate Committee should study how best the building could be used to further the aims of the College. A subcommittee was set up under the chairmanship of D. G. (Tim) Wilson,

> To consider the development of the College headquarters as an educational centre and, when requested, to carry out executive action in this matter.

This subcommittee included in its membership representatives of the other academic committees and of the metropolitan and Home Counties faculties. It was the precursor of the Headquarters Courses Committee.

In December 1963 Tim Wilson became Chairman of the Postgraduate Committee and it was appropriate that during his chairmanship the British Postgraduate Medical Federation invited the College to organize the first course to be held at Princes Gate under Section 63 of the NHS Act. This course, entitled 'Early Years in General Practice', took place on October 19–23 1964 and was the first course for which trainees were eligible for Ministry of Health grants.

Tim Wilson had to resign in April 1964 owing to ill health and was succeeded by W. (Bill) Hylton who had already given much help to the committee, particularly in the first part of Vocational Training. The committee recommended Council to establish a working party 'To investigate how the College can organize and help others to organize pre-practice Vocational Training for general practice'. This working party was set up under the chairmanship of Bill Hylton and was the forerunner of the Vocational Training Subcommittee.

By 1964 the Postgraduate Committee had become responsible for several tasks which could best be carried out by separate groups of people. These included the development of vocational training, the use of Princes

Gate as an educational centre, the development of continuing education in the postgraduate centres, the adjudication of awards and the medical recording service.

It had also become apparent that the separation of undergraduate from postgraduate education was artificial.

The Postgraduate Committee, which had existed since the College's second year, was abolished in January 1965, when its duties were taken over by the new Education Committee of Council.

PART II: 1965–1977

Donald Irvine

In the College's first 13 years many of its most active members were modernizing the structure and organization of their own practices, and set about securing diagnostic and treatment facilities for their work in hospitals. A number of them described their practices and the changes they had made so that other people could see what they were doing. Many of their ideas were adopted by other enthusiasts and so change began to snowball. At the same time, several outstanding individuals began to describe morbidity in their own practices and to lay the foundations for national morbidity surveys (see Chapter XI). Their work provided the first tangible evidence that the pattern of diseases and illnesses which general practitioners saw was significantly different from that encountered by their hospital colleagues. Furthermore, their data showed that about 90% of illness episodes were dealt with entirely by general practitioners.

The Medical Recording Service was doing well (see Chapter IX), bringing continuing education, including the new information about general practice, into doctors' homes and surgeries, often through listening groups. The proposal for postgraduate centres was still strongly supported. A start was made to try to give general practice a presence in the universities, and an examination was introduced by the College, after much argument and soul-searching, to set a standard in general practice.

THE CHARTER CRISIS

In the 1960s, in spite of all these activities, morale in general practice began to slide downwards again. Many practitioners resented the recent changes, for they liked the *status quo*. They could see no point in spending more time or money on so-called improvements. Others were frustrated because they were financially penalized for making their practices more efficient. Some emigrated; but others began to fight hard for a better deal and they were, in the main, successful.

Lessons for the College

The events leading to the Charter Agreement (1966) had first and foremost shown the necessity of documenting the work of general practice. Armed with facts, the medical politicians could argue a better case. They showed that new ideas could be introduced in general practice provided that enough successful examples could be put into operation first by a reasonably sized minority of enthusiasts. They reminded the College that BMA support was essential to complete the process of change on a national scale and they revealed that government would provide new money for general practice if it was to be used to improve the service for patients. For the College the Charter was merely an important step forwards, not an end in itself. It had produced new resources and facilities and put new life into general practice. It did not ask anything of the doctors themselves. Thus the problem of defining the work of general practice, and about the equipment a doctor would require to carry this out properly, remained virtually untouched.

The College had a powerful incentive to work these questions out. Their solution was fundamental to a true internal renewal in general practice. Despite the Charter, the College concluded, the future was still far from certain.

VOCATIONAL TRAINING FOR GENERAL PRACTICE

In the late 1960s, the College's decision to focus its main educational effort on vocational training had been shaped by several factors. Firstly, vocational training was needed urgently. Secondly, there were the lessons of the Charter events. Thirdly, the College's earliest attempts to introduce general practice as a subject in its own right into the universities had, with one or two exceptions, ended in failure. In the 1960s even some of the most informed practitioners, when pressed, were unable to explain satisfactorily to their university colleagues how their clinical work might contribute uniquely to basic medical education. The fourth factor was the recent failure of the trainee general practitioner scheme. The trainee year, introduced by government and the BMA in the early 1950s, had been a good idea which had fallen into disrepute and then collapsed for several reasons. The manpower crisis made it easy for a young doctor to find a practice without preliminary experience under supervision. Training practices, selected by local medical committees, were too often of poor quality, and misused their trainees. The trainee year had been regarded as an opportunity mainly to learn about practice finance and organization. Young doctors fresh from hospital knew much about scientific clinical medicine, often more than their teachers; general practice had virtually nothing more to offer them in that respect. And lastly, there was no agreed theme and no organization; everybody went their own way.

A Fresh Start

Systematic vocational training seemed to be ideal for a new start. It would give time to think more carefully about the content and nature of general practice, to work out how it could be assessed realistically, and perhaps give some clues about how continuing education and the teaching of medical students should develop in future. It should be possible to show medical students what general practice had to offer as a clinical subject if young doctors were placed with carefully chosen general practitioners who had respectable clinical reputations and who wanted to take teaching seriously. Since this vocational training was specifically for general practice, it would not challenge the specialists on their own ground or compete for their resources. And because it would be for a short period of time, and involve relatively small numbers of young doctors, the logistics could be manageable. Lastly, the use in the early stages of volunteer trainees and trainers who were known to be really enthusiastic about their work, coupled with thorough planning and organization, should provide the optimum conditions to find out whether the College's basic ideas about good practice were sound or not.

Early Plans

Thus the foundations were laid and by 1965 the Education Committee of Council had been created. The College had formed a working party in 1964 'to investigate how it could organize, and help others to organize, pre-practice vocational training for general practice from the date of qualification'. The Report on *Special Vocational Training for General Practice*[9] was published in 1965. In 1966 the College put forward detailed, carefully thought out, evidence to Lord Todd's Royal Commission on Medical Education setting out the reasons why general practice was a subject in its own right, the case for departments of general practice, vocational training and better continuing education. It was a far-sighted document, for it broke new ground by anticipating some of the radical changes needed in medical education as a whole. A further paper[10] on the implementation of vocational training followed in 1967. Thus, in the hopeful anticipation of a favourable Royal Commission Report, the College laid its plans as thoroughly as it could. The senior members responsible had by this time recruited a number of younger principals to their cause. These men and women were eager to help and to learn, and were prepared to become responsible for the organization of field trials.

The Todd Commissions's Report[11], when it appeared in 1968, was everything the College could have wished for.

Theory into Practice

The working parties which had done the preliminary thinking were replaced in 1968 by the *College's Vocational Training Subcommittee*. For seven years this subcommittee became the nerve centre for general practice vocational training. Its job was to help find solutions to problems as they arose in the experimental schemes and, in general, to act as a fast communications system and forum for ideas for all those most intimately involved. It was highly successful in fulfilling these functions. The younger members who were starting, or had already started, schemes in Wessex, North-east England, Thames Valley, East Anglia, Kent and Northern Ireland were brought into continuing and close contact with each other and with the central operation. They were urged to try out their own ideas since nobody knew 'a best way'. Arrangements were made to monitor the results of their work by the Department of General Practice in Manchester. The General Medical Services Committee of the BMA (GMSC) was asked to help at an early stage, as a crop of unforeseen problems involving new finance and terms and conditions of service were encountered. Soon after, the College joined with the GMSC and the Health Departments to form a *Standing Working Group* which could handle these problems with the minimum of delay.

The early years of vocational training were exciting, for everyone involved felt they were breaking new ground. College members had thrown everything they had into the early schemes because they knew that their College's own ideas were now on trial.

Contents and Aims of Training

It soon became obvious that more help was needed by scheme organizers and trainers who were still not quite sure what they were trying to teach or how best to do it. A small working party appointed by the College dealt quickly with the most urgent problems about organizing training. Its first report was published in 1971. The main report, *The Future General Practitioner: Learning and Teaching*[12], was a major work intended for trainers in general practice. Published in 1972, it was a milestone even though it was controversial then and is still. Its object was to draw together what was known of the clinical content of general practice and to link this with the work of the general-practice team. A working job definition for the future general practitioner was agreed, from which educational aims were derived. Five main areas of content were described. General practice was presented as a clinical discipline which could be taught and learnt largely in general practice. Here was a carefully constructed thesis, based on the results of research done in general practice which others could use, adapt, modify and improve. Once again people close to the scene felt they could refute the specialists' claim that general practice was simply the sum of a number of specialties practised at a fairly superficial level.

The College was no longer defending the concept of general practice as a discipline in itself; in the realm of ideas it was now going on to the offensive. The general concept appeared to have made sense although some people argued fiercely about the details. In a slightly modified form the working definition and the educational aims were presented by the Leeuwenhorst Group to all important bodies concerned with vocational training in Europe. These modified aims are now the basis for vocational training for general practice in the United Kingdom and the European Economic Community.

The College also worked closely with other Royal Colleges and Faculties to describe certain aspects of those specialist subjects which were most relevant to general practice. There have been joint publications with the Royal College of Physicians, the Royal College of Obstetricians and Gynaecologists and with the Royal College of Psychiatrists. The College's publication with the British Paediatric Association was later reproduced in full as an appendix to the Court Report[13]. More recently the College and the British Geriatric Association have described the needs of the future general practitioner in the care of the elderly. An expert working party was examining preventive medicine and its place in general practice.

Lastly, the College continued to refine and develop its philosophy for the future of general practice in medicine in two very thoroughly prepared papers – the Evidence to the Merrison Committee on *The Regulation of the Medical Profession* and the Evidence to the Royal Commission on the National Health Service.

Teaching in General Practice

General practice, unlike the specialties, has little tradition of teaching because for a long while it had been almost excluded from this activity in medical schools (see Chapter VII). In the event there were advantages in starting from scratch. It was possible to look at disciplines outside medicine, especially those concerned with the behavioural sciences, to see what could be usefully assimilated and used in general practice. It meant also that general practice could work out methods which were most appropriate for doctors who were used to working on their own and who, as a result, did not have the regular, informal stimulus of daily contact with colleagues. Time for teaching was fundamental. A variety of one-to-one teaching methods suitable for use in the practice were developed, and the immense value of small group teaching for trainers and trainees was established unequivocally. It was surprising how quickly these methods were accepted and absorbed into general practice. It was encouraging to see how they helped trainers and trainees to lay out their work for inspection by their peers, to become self-critical and to learn how to become critical of others without giving offence.

The College placed clinical quality first in the choice of trainers and teaching practices, although this was not always successful in the event. Nevertheless, it introduced academic criteria in the selection of trainers for the first time. Not surprisingly this approach involved, and still does, choosing trainers, if necessary by invitation, who are recognized as good clinicians and teachers. Despite difficulties, the criteria required by the College have been adopted by the Joint Committee on Postgraduate Training for General Practice (JCPTGP) and the regional postgraduate committees. However, there are wide variations in the way in which they are interpreted and applied, revealing the underlying differences in attitudes.

The value of visiting posts in training schemes was first suggested by experience with the inspections carried out by the Royal College of Physicians and our College jointly on junior hospital medical posts. The College introduced its own programme of visiting training practices which had asked for College recognition in 1975. The methods developed for these visits were adapted and refined by the JCPTGP, which carried out the inspections for its own purposes and on behalf of the College.

The Nuffield Course

Although training went well in the experimental schemes, it became clear in the early 1970s that the rapid expansion needed elsewhere in the country might not happen successfully unless new local leaders could be prepared for their work. The College invited the Nuffield Provincial Hospitals Trust and the Health Departments to finance an ambitious course in order to help fill this gap. About 100 doctors attended one of the three courses at Princes Gate. The Nuffield Course[14] was criticized for its methods, which drew heavily on educational theory. Nevertheless the courses succeeded in their primary aim because they helped course organizers to understand themselves and general practice better, and how to help others to learn to teach. It appeared that the doctors chosen have in turn influenced many trainers, and the whole operation provided a momentum just when it was needed.

Organization

Vocational training introduced an educational structure for general practice. Regional advisers, associate regional advisers, course organizers, College tutors and trainers were gradually being brought together in integrated organizations based on the regional postgraduate institutes. College personnel in the experimental and later schemes played a key role in identifying the jobs to be done and the kind of appointments necessary to carry them out.

Assessment and Standards

The MRCGP examination soon became the normal pathway to membership of the College (see Chapter X).

Trainees

The College has listened carefully to what trainees have said and thought about the nature and quality of their training. Trainee general practitioners have been involved in the organization of the best schemes to a far greater extent than have junior hospital doctors in theirs. The College kept itself informed of trainee opinion by organizing three national conferences.

Postgraduate Training Subcommittee for General Practice

In 1975, as it became clear that vocational training was going to be introduced for all future principals, the College replaced the Vocational Training Subcommittee with a new committee of Council, *The Postgraduate Training Committee*.

101

The Future

During the past 25 years the College has emerged to become an organization of real significance in education for general practice. Today it is the academic headquarters for general practice. It sets a national standard through its membership examination. It has acquired a substantial influence on the whole of medical education largely as a result of its single-minded and sustained efforts in vocational training.

References

1. College of General Practitioners (1957–1958). Continuing education of general practioners. An analysis of replies to a questionnaire from the Postgraduate Education Committee of Council. *Research Newsletter* **NS4**, 151–152, 242–249, 329–334; *J. Coll. Gen. Practit.*, **I**, 36–41, 171–175, 262–264
2. College of General Practitioners (1956). Conference on General Practitioner Obstetrics. *Research Newsletter* **NS3**, No. 1, Suppl.
3. College of General Practitioners (1956). Report on the conference on some practical aspects of postgraduate work in the faculties of the College. *Research Newsletter*, **NS3**, 118–130.
4. Cranbrook Report (1959). *Report of the Maternity Services Committee.* Ministry of Health. (London: HMSO)
5. College of General Practitioners (1956). Memorandum on general-practitioner maternity services. *Research Newsletter*, **NS3**, 175–182
6. College of General Practitioners (1961). Emotional disorders in general practice. *J. Coll. Gen. Practit.*, **4**, Suppl., 2
7. College of General Practitioners (1959). Memorandum for the guidance of trainers. *J. Coll. Gen. Practit.*, **2**, Suppl., 1
8. College of General Practitioners (1961). Opportunities for Postgraduate Education. A Report on the Postgraduate Questionnaire of February 1960. *J. Coll. Gen. Practit.*, **4**, 318–322
9. College of General Practitioners (1965). *Special vocational training for general practice.* Reports from General Practice I. (London: CGP)
10. College of General Practitioners (1967). *The Implementation of Vocational Training.* Reports from General Practice 6. (London: CGP)
11. Todd Report (1968). *Royal Commission on Medical Education 1965–68.* Report. (London: HMSO)
12. Royal College of General Practitioners (1972). *The Future General Practitioner. Learning and Teaching.* (London: British Medical Journal)
13. Court Report (1976). *Fit for the Future.* Report of the Committee on Child Health Services. (London: HMSO)
14. Freeling, P. and Barry, S. (1982). *In-Service Training.* A Study of the Nuffield Courses of the Royal College of General Practitioners. (Windsor: NFER-Nelson)

IX
THE MEDICAL RECORDING SERVICE AND THE MEDICAL AUDIOVISUAL LIBRARY

John* and Valerie Graves

This is the story of an enterprise that started as a College activity, grew like a cuckoo in the nest (to the surprise and sometimes dismay of its parents) and eventually became an independent organization.

In the 1950s the young College abounded in members stung by the Collings Report, irritated by 'Moran's ladder', and frustrated by inadequate courses and training, who wanted to prove themselves. One of them was John Graves, in 1955 a very junior partner in semi-rural practice. His wife, Valerie, with a background of academic medical research but then tied by four small children, had looked in vain for work to do at home. The College provided it: Robin Pinsent and Ian Watson needed help with the Measles Survey, providing contact with over 100 enthusiastic members. Next she handled the College's 1955/56 questionnaire to all members, giving access to information about general practitioners' frustrations and needs, such as lack of opportunity for appropriate study.

Why not, therefore, take courses to the doctor in his own home, if he could not find what he wanted outside? John and Valerie picked 50 members from the questionnaire replies, asking if they would take part in a pilot trial of educational material for home study. Twenty-seven agreed. Smith, Kline and French Laboratories Ltd financed the trial, Robin Pinsent and George Swift acted as catalysts. Talks were recorded on tape and long-playing discs, listeners sent them round to one another to save postage (the

---

* John Graves died on January 17 1980.

'listening circuits'). Early topics included 'virus disease', 'psychiatry in general practice', 'are colds catching?', and 'the death certificate'.

In 1958 John, travelling with an Upjohn Fellowship, collected more enthusiasts, some from isolated country areas but also from large towns like Glasgow and Birmingham, where academic isolation was often worse. An article in the *British Medical Journal*[1] in September 1958 produced enormous interest from doctors in hospital and overseas as well as more general practitioners. The College agreed to continue the project, which became known as the Medical Recording Service, reporting to the Post-graduate Education Committee of Council but run by John and Valerie from their own home.

The pattern in the early years was to make six recordings, with slides, each year for the circuits: a kind of magazine service, topics being chosen to promote discussion – new concepts rather than new drugs. Listeners did not know what they would hear, which encouraged them to keep an open mind. Topics of less general appeal (heart sounds, or hypnosis) were not sent round the circuits but lent on request – the beginnings of the library which eventually dominated the service. Talks were specially commissioned: recordings made at meetings were rarely popular.

Who listened? In 1960 there were 285 circuit members (rising to 450 later), youngish, enthusiastic College members, some of whom later became active in the postgraduate centre movement, in vocational training and in university departments. They ran small discussion groups (of partners, local colleagues, district nurses, consultants) to listen to tapes over beer and sandwiches and to argue far into the night. They could record comments and questions and the speaker would reply. Discussion groups were a great success: they brought good speakers right into the doctor's home and also brought people together to teach themselves. They created a desire for learning and a demand for high standards of teaching. (As organized courses improved, circuits were needed less. They stopped in 1965.)

During the 1960s the circuit discussion groups were a valued benefit of College membership, and helped to enhance the College's reputation for innovation and enthusiasm. There were stories of partnerships between rival single-handed general practitioners starting from a tape group, and of out-of-date consultants being gently coaxed to try new ideas. At the same time the lending library side of the Recording Service was growing – 5000 loans in 1965. It was used by some general practitioners who were not members of the College – nurses, doctors in public health, hospital, in industry and overseas. A tape could go 'anywhere in the world for a shilling' in those days: they went to Australia, Burma, Ethiopia, Fiji, Israel, Rhodesia, South Africa, Sudan, Sweden and the West Indies. This brought the College's name, as a pioneer in educational technology, to far-flung people and places;to reach a mission hospital in Peru, tapes travelled by plane, rail, river boat and finally by llama. A College official bringing (he thought) the first message to Iceland found a College tape on his host's mantelpiece.

At this time John and Valerie were involved in other College activities – Postgraduate Education Committee, Vocational Training Working Party, Headquarters Courses Subcommittee. Valerie ran 'Early Years' and 'Trainers' Courses' for many years and saw general practitioners becoming acceptable as course speakers and organizers – a novel idea then. (There was great antagonism to Balint-oriented teaching: one postgraduate dean objected – 'But Dr Graves, you cannot really believe that a state of mind can produce a symptom?') They worked with, for example, the BMA Film Committee, the *British Medical Journal*, the Royal Society of Medicine General Practice Section, the Association for the Study of Medical Education, and the British Broadcasting Corporation on the television series for doctors 'Medicine Today'. In this way they built up a wide circle of contacts and potential speakers. Valerie became a general-practitioner principal herself in 1964 and gradually had less time for committee work.

The Medical Recording Service was helped by grants from Smith, Kline and French Ltd until 1968. By then much of its income came from loan charges to non-members. In 1963 tapes on smallpox, made urgently for the Ministry of Health at the time of an epidemic, were very successful. Encouraged by A. Talbot Rogers and later by George Godber, the Ministry (later the Department of Health and Social Security) supported the Medical Recording Service with grants for many years.

Until 1962 John and Valerie ran the Service entirely themselves, doing the artwork, photography, recording, copying, despatch of tapes and correspondence. Mrs Freda Reed (librarian) and Mrs Fay Fontana (secretary, later administrator) came to help in 1962. As the work expanded more staff were taken on – a cottage industry gradually acquiring higher standards of equipment and skilled technicians. Mrs Barbara Trevor became librarian in 1968. The work spread from room to room of the Graves' rambling Victorian house (Kitts Croft, at Writtle, near Chelmsford).

Some of the most popular tapes for general practitioners were symptom based, such as 'It's my eye, doctor' or 'It's my skin, doctor', but basic science tapes, like 'Sodium and Water Metabolism', interested general practitioners as well as hospital doctors. Ephemeral subjects like 'NHS Reorganization' were particularly suitable for tape-slide. Other popular series were 'Anaesthetics for Nurses', 'Educating and Training the Mentally Handicapped' (for subnormality nurses) and 'Handling the Cerebral Palsy Child' (for remedial therapists).

The Service co-operated with many academic organizations, such as the British Orthopaedic Association, Association of Clinical Pathologists, Royal College of Obstetricians and Gynaecologists (which later set up its own tape library) and the Royal College of Surgeons, to produce series of tape-slides for planned and defined postgraduate needs. John and Valerie had always hoped that they would be asked to work with their own College, but a need for tape-slides was never felt, though a working party with the North-west England faculty to assess tapes for vocational training was set up in 1976.

Long-playing discs were stopped in 1965 and reel-to-reel tapes in 1978 in favour of cassettes. Most tapes had accompanying slides. There were slide sets with printed commentaries, for instance, on 'First-aid (common injuries)', 'Common Infectious Diseases', Parasites' etc, and on aspects of community health, made with a Nuffield Provincial Hospitals Trust grant in 1971/72. Recordings of heart and chest sounds, voices and interviews with patients, were included. Tapes could be used by individuals at home or in a library (using headphones), for small group study. Tape-slide equipment began to be installed in hospital and medical school libraries.

It was always a personal service by John and Valerie for their listeners; newsletters kept up the personal touch. Visitors from all over the world came to Kitts Croft to see how tape-slides were made. Conferences were held in 1963, 1967 and 1970, and in 1967 John visited the USA on a Commonwealth Foundation Fellowship, meeting old friends and seeing tape-slides and videotape in use there.

By 1969 John and Valerie (prompted by the College Auditor, Ancrum Evans) were becoming anxious about the legal and financial status of the Service. It had no real existence, but had a large cash turnover, expensive equipment and wages to pay for eight staff. Should it become a private company, separate from the College? Some Council members were not sure whether the College ought to be involved in what almost amounted to an industry. Though uneasy about the Service making money and perhaps altering the College's charitable status, Council were equally alarmed that it might run into debt. So, by Special Resolution at the General Meeting in Cambridge, April 1969, a Foundation was set up.

The Medical Recording Service Foundation Board met, usually twice a year, from 1970. Its first members were A. Talbot Rogers (Chairman), John Graves (Secretary), Jack Lord (Treasurer – one of the early circuit members), Dame Annis Gillie (Chairman of the Foundation's first Committee), Professor Kenneth Hill (Professor of Pathology, Royal Free Hospital, interested in developing countries), Professor John Anderson (Professor of Medicine, King's College Hospital, interested in under-graduate teaching), Valerie Graves, George Swift and Patrick Byrne (representing the College), Miss Winifred Hector (lately Senior Nursing Tutor, St Bartholomew's Hospital School of Nursing), Ronald McG. Harden (from Glasgow, later to be Professor of Medical Education at Dundee) and Bryce Stewart (observer from the Department of Health and Social Security).

In 1970, output reached 15 000 loans and sales, many going overseas but half still to general practitioners. 1971 was a year of crisis, a prolonged postal strike causing six weeks' loss of income – highlighting anxiety about money – the Service having no capital reserve. A work study and a cost accounting survey were set up, introducing Mr Harold Ansell of Pike Russell Ltd, whose advice helped the Service through many crises. He recommended sharply increased charges: 60p to College members (previously free) and £1 to others. This did not cause output to drop: analysis showed increased use by nurses and junior hospital staff, encouraged by the new trend of distributing tapes made by other people, such as the Universities of Glasgow and Newcastle. General practitioners were no longer the principal users but they were still the largest single group. Circuits had stopped five years previously, though general practitioners still ran some home discussion groups.

In 1972 the College became 'Royal'. John Graves took photographs and recordings of Prince Philip's visit. (Recordings of College archives, personalities and occasions had been made since 1957.) On November 1 1972, the James Mackenzie lecture was recorded and, at the College Dinner given that evening at the Grosvenor House for about 800 people, so were the speeches, including those by Lord Todd and HRH The Prince Philip, Duke of Edinburgh.

At Kitts Croft, the first Open Day – the first of many happy occasions – was held in June 1972. There were now 14 staff including a professionally qualified recording technician, artist and photographer. A fully-equipped recording studio was installed at 14 Princes Gate. The Service was making tapes on a wide variety of topics and for many and diverse educational institutions. A monumental series on 'Developmental Paediatrics', for many years among the library's 'top pops', was being made with Mary Sheridan, John Graves taking photographs, Valerie demonstrating assessments on her own patients. For years a new Sheridan tape was certain of immediate demand from community physicians and health visitors.

1973 saw a big expansion with output at 20 000. A co-operative venture with several medical schools was started, called MASPA (Medical Audio-tape Slide Producers' Association) for the exchange of tapes between schools. Dr Kenneth Easton of Catterick contributed tapes to the thriving collection on first-aid and road smash rescue, and the 'top pop' topic was 'Problem Orientated Medical Records'. Sadly, Professor Kenneth Hill died;

he was replaced by Professor David Morley, paediatrician and founder of TALC (Teaching Aids at Low Cost), which produced slides and tapes on child health for developing countries. Talbot Rogers retired in 1974 because of ill health and Sir George Godber became chairman.

Was the Medical Recording Service Foundation (MRSF) still appropriate for the College in 1974? Not now so much needed by College members, it was expanding rapidly elsewhere. 1975 was a year of terrible financial cutback throughout the National Health Service but, thanks to its now efficient cost accounting and to large overseas sales, the MRSF remained solvent and started a capital fund. A working party discussed these issues, including the need for a permanent home for the library; it was outgrowing Kitts Croft and could never feel secure while dependent on John and Valerie. One of the Chelmsford hospitals had offered a site. The working party also agreed on wider aims for the Service – other media, such as videotape, and more work for medical schools. A full-time travelling representative to assist Mrs Fontana, Mrs Brokenbrow, had been appointed in 1973 and in 1975 Miss Myrtle Marshall took her place. John and Valerie visited medical schools to promote MASPA, which was flourishing. The 'top-pop' topic was 'Non-accidental Injury'.

Surveys in 1974 and 1975 showed nurses and junior hospital staff to be the largest users of the loan service. General practitioners now made up only 20%. Sales were chiefly to medical schools in the UK and overseas. Output in 1975 was 28 000.

In 1976 anxiety about the relationship of the MRSF to the College came to a head with Ancrum Evans doubting whether its activities came within the College's registered charitable aims, now that it made tapes, for example, for dentists or overseas medical schools. If not, its income would be liable to Corporation Tax. It became clear that forming the Foundation had not given the Service any independent structure – it was still part of the College. Eventually, the opinion of Counsel (Mr Robert Walker) was sought in January 1977. He recommended either a trading company within the College (to covenant income back to the parent, as was done by many charities) or an independent charity.

John and Valerie would have liked the Service to remain within the College, but College Council did not wish to keep it as a trading company, so separation was inevitable. It was an especially sad moment because July 1977 was the twentieth anniversary of their long association with the College as pioneers of a new style of teaching – not just the technology of tape-slide but of self-help and small-group learning. The College's name would no longer be heard on every tape.

The new charity was set up in November 1977 – 25 years after the College was born – and was called the Graves Medical Audiovisual Library.

It would still use the studio at 14 Princes Gate, allow cheap rates to College members, and have College representatives on its new Council of management, but inevitably in the future the links with the College would weaken.

After many frustrations, the hospital site was abandoned. An old house in Chelmsford (Holly House, 220 New London Road) was bought in 1977 and extensively reconstructed. The Library moved there in May 1978, and an assistant medical director (Peter Leatherdale) was appointed to help John and Valerie. It was a splendid home for the new Graves Library – looking backwards to the Royal College of General Practitioners but forwards to an independent future.

Reference

1.   Graves, J. C. and Graves, V. (1958). Keeping informed by tape and disk. *Br. Med. J.,* **ii**, 583–585

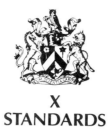

X
STANDARDS

PART I

THE CRITERIA COMMITTEE

William S. Gardner

The problem of criteria for membership of the College was discussed by the Steering Committee which determined that the College should not be merely, in Guy Ollerenshaw's words, a 'Chums' Club'. It knew that strict academic standards for membership would, in the end, be needed. But it was necessary to start in a small way.

Foundation Membership

The Provisional Foundation Council recommended that Foundation Membership should be restricted to those whose names were on *The Medical Register* and who had joined the College as members before the first Annual General Meeting on November 14 1953 and who had been:

(1) Twenty years in general practice or its equivalent as a general medical officer (with primary charge of patients) in a school, factory or similar institution, in Her Majesty's Forces, Colonial Medical Service, Merchant Navy etc;

or (2) Five years in general practice (or its equivalent) and who gave an undertaking to accept postgraduate instruction for three days (or a corresponding number of hours) each year, or for five and a half days every two years;

or   (3) Five years in general practice (or its equivalent) and who possessed a higher postgraduate degree or diploma.

During the first three weeks 1077 members enrolled. 142 other doctors who were unable to fulfil the recommended criteria for foundation membership joined as Foundation Associates.

Foundation Associateship

Associateship was intended to encourage, interest and involve in the work of the College younger doctors who intended to devote their careers to general practice, and to help them in their progress to full membership. Others, working in specialist disciplines but who were interested in general practice and in our developing College, and who were anxious to be of assistance, could also join by becoming Associates.

Foundation Membership (MCGP)

The full Foundation Council on April 18 1953 endorsed the decision of the Provisional Foundation Council, that the time was not yet ripe for members to use the letters MCGP after their names. However, the Editor of *The Medical Directory* agreed to enter details of the College and its officers on the appropriate collegiate page, and to an entry of the words 'Foundation Member (or Associate) of the College of General Practitioners' in the practitioner's personal entry relating to learned societies.

Before the College was six months old, more than 2000 doctors had joined it, 130 of whom were from overseas.

The first Annual General Meeting resolved that the question of criteria for Associateship and Membership be considered by Council during the ensuing year. To implement this decision, a Criteria Committee of Council was formed on January 20 1954, with J. G. Ollerenshaw as Chairman and J. Cotterell honorary secretary.

It was considered that the views of the whole membership of the College should be obtained. A questionnaire was sent to each faculty and the replies were helpful for future planning.

Criteria for full Associateship

The agreed criteria for full Associateship were:

(1) The acceptance of an associate be automatic on receipt of an

application form and such entrance fee or annual subscription as may be determined.

(2) A person shall be eligible for admission as an associate if he
  (a) (i) is a registered medical practitioner, or
      (ii) is a qualified medical practitioner during his period of provisional registration. Any person so admitted shall cease to be an associate if he fails to obtain registration within two years of qualification.
  (b) gives an undertaking that he continues approved postgraduate study if he enters and remains in active general practice and that he will uphold and promote the aims of the College to the best of his ability.

Criteria for full Membership

Whatever the criteria, it was fundamental that they ensured that successful applicants were providing good service to their patients and were prepared to maintain high standards. There were many types of general practice, and the versatility of general practitioners made it necessary to accept a wide variety of qualities and attributes. Many criteria were suggested and all received careful consideration. No single one could be devised which would invariably admit to Membership. After deliberation the following recommendations were made and agreed by Council as our first criteria for full membership:

(1) That applicants for membership should submit to Council evidence of all their medical activities over as wide a range as possible and that this evidence should be considered as a whole by a Board of Censors.

(2) That those who are already members should not be called upon to submit such evidence or make any new application.

(3) That membership should not be restricted to principals.

(4) That the same criteria apply for membership overseas as for that in the British Isles.

(5) That bye-law 5 should read:
  (a) A person shall be eligible to apply for admission as a member of the College if he
      (i) is a registered medical practitioner who has been qualified for not less than seven years;

    (ii) is proposed and seconded by two members of the College, these sponsors not being in partnership with each other;

    (iii) has been engaged in general practice either for a minimum period of five years or for a minimum period of three years as an associate of the College.

(b) An applicant for membership must satisfy the Council of the College of the high standard of his work in general practice by:

    (i) evidence submitted by the applicant himself, on an application form, concerning his practice, experience, and. academic and administrative achievements;

    (ii) supporting evidence obtained by the Council from the applicant's sponsors, the board of his faculty or others whom he or his sponsors have chosen to appoint.

(c) An applicant must also

    (i) submit himself to an interview with the censors, if required;

    (ii) give an undertaking that he will continue approved post-graduate study while he remains in active general practice, and that he will uphold and promote the aims of the College to the best of his ability.

As with associateship, an undertaking to continue postgraduate study was an essential part of membership.

Seniority

As membership of the College should indicate a practitioner of mature and balanced judgement, a period of seven years after registration before membership could be applied for was thought to be suitable.

Sponsors

Sponsorship was not to be undertaken lightly. Certain difficulties arose as a result of this regulation. For example, doctors working in isolated areas could not always find two sponsors who had enough experience of the candidate's methods to comment upon them. Separate and confidential 'sponsor forms' in the name of each applicant were prepared. These were of much assistance, especially when attempting to assess the position of doctors from sparsely populated regions.

The Application Form

This was carefully designed in order to allow the candidate scope to describe his practice, its organization, his academic experience, and the work he may have done for the College. Important items included postgraduate studies, hospital appointments, research work in general practice, teaching of general practice, involvement in medical societies and associations, and published work.

Supporting Evidence

Supporting evidence was required by Council in addition to the information already given on the application form. Usually, most of this additional information came from the faculty board in the applicant's area of practice. Even at local level unforeseen problems came to light. For example, no member of a board might know the applicant or the quality of his work. This was frequently the case in isolated practices; but even in urban areas the preference of some doctors to work in isolation made this reporting unsatisfactory.

Report of Criteria Committee of Council

The committee reported to Council on July 21 1954. Its recommendations about criteria for associateship and membership were accepted. The committee recommended the appointment of a Board of Censors.

THE BOARD OF CENSORS

John Burdon, John Fry, William S. Gardner

Every application for membership to the new Board of Censors was accompanied by a suitable dossier, which needed much time and effort to look through. It was recommended to Council that this Board should consist of ten members, including two from each of the undergraduate, postgraduate and research committees.

The Board of Censors was officially approved at the second Annual General Meeting of the College (1954). Its terms of reference were:

To advise and assist Council on questions concerned with applications for Membership and Associateship of the College.

115

Its first chairman was J. G. Ollerenshaw, vice-chairman R. M. S. McConaghey and honorary secretary J. H. Hunt. In its search for a method of assessment of candidates, without a formal examination, the Board had many difficult decisions in the preparation of application forms, the supervision of the bye-laws (particularly as they referred to applicants from overseas) and other matters such as the need for two sponsors, reports from faculty boards and interviews with applicants. The first bye-laws were based on their early experiences.

The Bye-laws

The bye-laws concerning associateship and membership engendered much discussion and thought. Council and the Criteria Committee asked for advice from numerous sources – from the Royal Medical Colleges, from faculties, from interested individuals, and from our College Solicitor, John Mayo. The word 'examination' kept infiltrating Council and Criteria Committee discussions. Feelings were deeply, and fairly evenly, divided on this subject. The conclusion of the first Council on this question was that the time was not yet ripe for introducing a formal examination as one of the criteria for membership. Arguments for and against were published in the Second *Annual Report*[1]. There was much debate both in Council and in the Criteria Committee. It was a matter which could not be agreed upon at this early stage in the development of the College. Two powerful opponents of examinations were George Abercrombie (Chairman of Council) and Guy Ollerenshaw (Chairman of the Criteria Committee and of the Board of Censors), both of whom made impassioned speeches at a Council meeting, which must have influenced members of Council who were undecided. Therefore other methods of assessment were developed by the Board of Censors.

Interviews with candidates at College headquarters or in faculties

There was a friendly, informal atmosphere at interviews with candidates. R. M. S. McConaghey, when he was chairman, always spoke quietly and showed great consideration. His often-penetrating questions evoked informative answers; but clinical matters were not touched upon. Basic facts about practice circumstances were elicited; and interest was shown in applicants' difficulties, leisure activities and the reasons why they wished to join the College. Motivation was regarded as highly important. Occasionally it became apparent that the applicant had come to criticize the College and its presumptions. One such lady with psychiatric leanings gave the Board a large piece of her mind in no uncertain terms, stamping out of the room without ceremony at the end of her attack. The question which had preceded this tirade had been quite inoffensive.

Interviews at the candidate's place of work

One method which was tried was to interview the applicant at his practice. This created many problems. It was costly and time-consuming. John Henderson from Pitlochry and William S. Gardner from Glasgow had on one occasion interviewed candidates in Dundee, Crieff and Lanarkshire. Fortunately the practices visited were first-class and the question of poor reports did not arise. However, these interviews at the practitioners' places of residence did bring to light difficulties involving distances and travelling, and the arranging of meetings. At that time, many doctors practised from their own homes, where the interviewers received generous hospitality and sometimes it proved difficult to fail a candidate under those circumstances.

Clinical assessment

Dissatisfaction was felt at a lack of clinical assessment. But the Board continued to try to identify doctors with strong motivation, who would persevere in the pursuit of the College's aims.

Written evidence

Most of the evidence about candidates was obtained from application forms on which facts were recorded, and from confidential reports from sponsors. Faculty honorary secretaries were also asked for comments. These forms grew more detailed, and the Board increasingly asked for interviews. By 1961 it was necessary to bring in 18 senior representatives from faculties to supplement the Board's numbers so that extra interviewing groups could run concurrently. Council reduced the work of the Board of Censors by delegating its power of admission of members. After another year the additional members of the Board numbered 22 and interviews were being asked for in every instance where the evidence had been insufficient.

In 1964 the Board was meeting at intervals of two or three months, and a screening committee of more experienced members sifted the applications, submitting for the Board's analysis only those which were not decided upon unanimously. This helped to ease the meetings, and made a drastic reduction in the Board's paper work.

The 1964 Questionnaire

In 1964 a questionnaire – a postal enquiry – was sent to all members on possible criteria for membership and brought in 3216 replies. These replies led to the development of a multiple-points system of assessment during 1965.

The multiple-points system of assessment

Several headings were identified. They included: Time spent in hospital junior appointments after registration (25 points). Time spent as a principal in general practice (50 points). Time spent as an assistant or trainee in general practice (25 points). Postgraduate degrees and diplomas (15 points). Submission of case reports with commentary, or other form of thesis (40 points). Time spent as a clinical assistant in hospital (15 points). Some test of knowledge of the details of clinical medicine and of the ancillary social services (40 points). Experience of special types of general practice in the armed forces, voluntary service overseas etc. (15 points). Research work (20 points). Submission of published papers (20 points). Attendance at postgraduate courses and other continuing education (20 points).

At the February 1965 meeting of the Board of Censors 216 applications were considered of which 209 were successful.

By 1966 the multiple-points system was in full swing, and censors were getting reasonably consistent results in their independent assessments; but the emphasis on 'objectivity' which the Board had adopted overshadowed other important considerations, so that less easily assessable qualities such as motivation, 'caritas', quality of premises, delegating ability, and 'general potential' received insufficient weight. Oral interviews were still needed, and sometimes practice visits by censors.

Long service in practice attracted 50 points. Associateship was rewarded by up to eight points (at two per year in practice); and the candidate could add points for innovations, practising obstetrics, being in charge of hospital beds, having teaching experience of vocational training and for well-organized and equipped premises.

A total of 400 points was available, though some criteria were mutually exclusive. Most young candidates obtained between 90 and 180, and the pass level was fixed at 120. It was clear that the failure rate could be arbitrarily raised at any time, but this idea was unpopular with the Board which, quite rightly, sought to refine its methods of assessment.

Assessors of written work

Nineteen assessors of written work were appointed, but their task was rendered difficult by the variety of work sent in, so that comparisons were impossible and a pass standard could not easily be decided.

When the examination became compulsory the points system automatically lapsed. The Board of Censors continued its function of appointing and supervising the examiners on Council's behalf, advising Council on matters pertaining to membership and encouraging and helping the work of the Examination Committee and Panel of Examiners.

PART II

THE EXAMINATION COMMITTEE

John F. Burdon, John Fry and William S. Gardner

The Second Council of the College had appointed an Examination Committee on December 15 1954, with the following terms of reference:

> To give full and detailed study to an examination as a possible method of entry to membership of the College of General Practitioners and to report to the Council of the College in 1955.

The chairman of this committee was F. M. Rose; J. M. Henderson was vice-chairman and W. S. Gardner honorary secretary.

The committee soon realized that it had a mammoth task and that it must work quickly. It considered the possibilities and value of conventional written examinations, case commentaries, theses, submission of published work, and clinical and oral examinations. The object of the proposed examination was to ensure that candidates had a good knowledge of the theory and technique of general medical practice, and that they were in touch with contemporary medical thought. It was appreciated that the range of the examination should be wide.

Few general practitioners had experience of organizing an examination. Much assistance was received from the Royal Colleges and the Royal Scottish Corporations, as well as from a number of individuals. It was clear that this examination should not be a repetition of the qualifying exams, nor one based on mere revision. Stress should be laid on the clinical and other aspects of general practice itself, such as practice organization, community medicine and human development.

The organization of the examination was discussed in great detail – where it should be held, its frequency, the appointment of examiners (with regulations for their guidance) and methods of marking and adjudication of results. A Panel of Advisers in Special Subjects was suggested, but this never materialized.

The submission of original work was considered to be a method of assessment acceptable to senior practitioners who might dislike the idea of a more formal type of examination. This could consists of case reports with commentary, a thesis or published work.

The Examination Committee reported to the College Council in March 1955 that:

(1) Such an examination was practicable, and
(2) It should consist, in its complete form, of written, clinical and oral tests. It should be for new members only. Submitted work should be assessed by the Board of Censors, should be optional, and if it were of a sufficiently high standard the candidate would be excused part or the whole of the examination.

This report was widely discussed; Council received it favourably, but did not commit itself to any immediate action.

Questionnaire to Faculties

All the faculties in the United Kingdom and overseas were contacted and asked to give their views on a possible examination for membership. The replies showed that there was a widespread feeling that the criteria for admission to membership were inadequate. The majority of faculties favoured the introduction of an examination. In particular, it was apparent that younger doctors felt that an examination for membership was necessary. These opinions were reported to the Fifth Council (1957)[2] and it was decided, in the meantime, to keep this question of an examination under constant review.

In 1959 the Examination Committee reported to Council again and suggested there should be a compulsory interview for all applicants for membership, a ceremony of admission to membership to be conducted by Provosts of faculties and the signing of a solemn declaration with regard to postgraduate study. Such ceremonies were to be conducted at faculty board meetings.

It recommended:

(1) An examination should be introduced as one of the criteria for entry to membership for those qualifying after March 31 1961.

(2) After March 31 1965 all applicants for membership should, except under special circumstances, either take the examination or submit written work.

The Examination Committee prepared a *Provisional Basis for a Syllabus and Guide for Future Candidates.* This was a comprehensive document in which were mentioned the clinical, technical, medico-legal and administrative subjects with which a general practitioner in the British Isles had to deal significantly often during his professional life. John Hunt had, in his own practice, kept records of the names of all the diseases and other problems with which he had to deal. This was the foundation of the syllabus to which all members of the committee contributed. This provisional syllabus also contained suggestions regarding the principles to be observed in framing the questions for the written paper, and sample papers were published in the report of the Examination Committee. Details regarding submitted work (case reports, a thesis or published work) were considered in lieu of, or in addition to, the results of an examination.

At the Seventh Annual General Meeting of the College (1960) the criteria for membership were discussed and the introduction of an examination was opposed by only a small majority. At that time the chairman of the Examination Committee was W. S. Gardner, vice-chairman R. Harkness, and honorary secretary J. F. Burdon.

In 1961 a most significant amendment to the terms of reference of the Examination Committee was passed:

To advise and assist Council in the introduction of an examination
as one of the criteria for membership or other grade of the College
to be taken into account by the Board of Censors.

These new terms of reference indicated a major change in the attitude of Council, faculties and members of the College towards an examination. Nearly all were agreed, now, that criteria for admission had to be strengthened; most younger doctors seemed to be insistent on this and were supporting an examination.

But in 1962 there occurred a recrudescence of the controversy surrounding the examination. A letter appeared in the *British Medical Journal* [3] from Professor Sir George Pickering, FRS, MD, FRCP, disapproving of the introduction of an examination for membership of our College. This initiated a correspondence in that journal which lasted for many weeks and included 45 letters.

Council's plans for an examination, and those of its Board of Censors and Examination Committee, went ahead. A *Court of Examiners* and *Working Party on the Administration of an Examination* were appointed.

121

THE EXAMINATION

John Fry and John H. Walker

The Court of Examiners

A Court of Examiners was appointed in 1965. The members were Lowell Lamont (chairman), J. D. E. Knox (honorary secretary), with L. W. Batten, P. S. Byrne, W. S. Gardner, Annis Gillie, J. H. Hunt and Richard Scott, and the Chairman of the Board of Censors *ex officio*.

Early Examinations

The examination was introduced gradually with only five candidates sitting the first examination on March 1 1965. The standard was high and all were successful. It was conducted entirely by general practitioners and consisted of written papers and an oral. For the following examination in May 1966 there were 15 candidates, all of whom were again successful. The Court was expanded at that time by the addition of E. V. Kuenssberg, R. J. F. H. Pinsent, George Swift and G. I. Watson. Paradoxically, this expansion was followed by a decline in the number of candidates, only 12 of whom attempted the examination during the academic year 1966/67.

In November 1967 the examination was cancelled through lack of support; but this temporary setback did not deter the Annual General Meeting, which decided that in future membership of the College should be achieved only by candidates who had completed a period of vocational training approved by Council (two years hospital work and two years in general practice), and had passed the Membership Examination. Prospective members were warned that this policy would be implemented in June 1968, for all except senior candidates who could submit satisfactory published work. The examination held in November that year attracted 32 candidates and, in May 1969, 46, establishing an upward trend which has continued.

Although the proposed Panel of Specialist Advisers was never established, the considerable academic problems involved in creating an examination in a subject as broad as general practice led the Court of Examiners to consult widely. The definition of the core content of vocational training, the role of the examination, its relationship to continuous assessment during training and the development of new and established examination techniques were all topics of concern to the Court and the Board of Censors. Close contact was established and maintained with the Australian College of General Practitioners, and considerable help was provided by the Royal College of Physicians.

Changes in the Examination

In 1968, a joint conference on examination techniques was held at the Royal College of Physicians[4], and was particularly notable for the fact that all present, including the Presidents of both Colleges, completed a multiple-choice question paper marked at the time and returned to the candidates. The success of this conference led to the inclusion of new techniques in the examination. A multiple-choice question paper (MCQ) of 200 questions was introduced. A modified-essay question paper (MEQ), designed to assess problem-solving abilities in general practice was devised, and an approach to the evaluation of the candidate's work in his own practice developed through the use of a Log Diary on 50 consecutive patients in his practice, in the first of the two oral examinations. The second oral examination was retained as an open-ended interview, and the traditional essay question paper (TEQ) was also retained, as a means of assessing candidates' skills in self-expression.

P.S. Byrne, the chairman of the Court of Examiners and Board of Censors, Keith Hodgkin and J. D. E. Knox played central roles in these developments. By 1970 the examination had assumed a format which, although its techniques were to be continually refined, was to remain largely unchanged for a decade.

The Court of Examiners was supplemented in 1968 by the appointment of a Panel of Additional Examiners. As the number of candidates began to rise, this panel was expanded. The problems of defining common standards within such a large group was approached by holding, in March 1970, the first of what was to become a regular series of Examiners' Conferences.

As well as discussing standards and the possible inclusion of new techniques, such as the simulated-patient interview (SPI), the panel was also able to consider the aims of the examination. In September 1971 these were defined as 'To test the competence of the ordinary general practitioner in his work'. At that time the Conference also considered the possible role of videotapes in the examination; it experimented with a clinical examination using patients; and it suggested ways in which the Log Diary could be improved. In a critical review of the techniques being used at that time it was concluded that factual recall was being adequately assessed by the multiple-choice question paper, attitudes and problem-solving by the modified essay, and the ability to marshal facts and present arguments by the traditional essay paper. While it was recognized that the wide range of behavioural, clinical and problem-solving skills required of the general practitioner might only be examined properly in a practice setting, the experiment using patients from general practice involved so many problems of validity and practicality that it was agreed that skills with patients should continue to be assessed by proxy in the oral examination. An approach to achieving uniformity of standards in the oral examination was begun through the use of experienced examiners as observers, commenting upon colleagues' technique and contributing to the assessment of borderline candidates.

During this period, all candidates were required to attend for oral examination. In 1973, however, it was appreciated that a group of candidates, whose marks in the written paper were so low as to place them beyond the possibility of success, were attending for oral examination unnecessarily. The Board of Censors therefore divided the examination into two parts, and only those candidates with reasonable marks in the written papers of Part I were invited to attend for orals.

Appointment of Examiners

The number of candidates continued to rise, and by 1975 had exceeded 400 a year. This inevitably produced increasing demands on examiners who, although appointed initially for a five-year period, were required often to serve much longer. Appointment to the Panel of Examiners was originally by invitation of the Chairman of the Court but, at this time, the procedure began to become more formalized. Members of the panel were nominated by faculties with the support of existing examiners; they were required to have passed the examination, to have attended a Study Day on its techniques, to be present at one of the Examiners' Workshops and to have observed one series of oral examinations. Appointed at the conclusion of this routine by the Board of Examiners, they served a probationary period of two years and were then appointed for a further five years.

The panel in 1977 consisted of 80 examiners. The conduct and development of the examination was the responsibility of an Examination Executive consisting of the Honorary Examination Secretary, four members appointed by the Board of Censors responsible for the individual components of the examination, and three members elected by the panel, with the Chairman of the Board of Censors and the Honorary Secretary of Council *ex officio*.

The organizational arrangements for the examination were considerable. The College was singularly fortunate in its staff and, in particular, it owes a considerable debt of gratitude to Mrs Pauline Dallmeyer who has been Executive Officer in charge of the Membership Department since 1971, the period during which the number of candidates rose from 100 to over 800 a year by 1977*.

---

* Editor's note: Four years later 1149 candidates applied to take the examination, of whom 739 were successful.

Review of the Aims of the Examination

The development of the examination coincided with the evolution of vocational training and, as the proportion of candidates sitting the examination on completion of the vocational training period increased, it became apparent that the original aim of the examination 'to test the competence of the ordinary general practitioner in his work' was no longer appropriate. The examiners therefore recommended to the Board of Censors that the aims of the examination should be revised and consist of:

> The assessment of the knowledge and competences appropriate to the general practitioner on completion of vocational training.

Content of Examination

The job definition of the general practitioner and the content of general practice had been defined in *The Future General Practitioner, Learning and Teaching*[5] and increasingly accepted as the basis of the examination. The explanatory notes for the MRCGP examination emphasized the five areas of knowledge to be assessed:

(1) *In Clinical Practice – Health and Disease* the candidate is required to demonstrate a knowledge of the diagnosis, management and, where appropriate, the prevention of diseases of importance in general practice.

(2) *In Human Development* he is expected to possess a knowledge of human development and demonstrate its value in the diagnosis and management of patients in general practice.

(3) *In Human Biology* he must demonstrate an understanding of human behaviour as it affects the presentation and management of disease in practice.

(4) *In Medicine and Society* the candidate must be familiar with common sociological and epidemiological concepts and their relevance to medical care, and demonstrate a knowledge of the organization of medical and related services in the United Kingdom and abroad.

(5) *In The Practice* the candidate must demonstrate a knowledge of good practice organization and be able to discuss recent developments in the evolution of general practice.

The College had accepted the educational objectives of the Working Party of the Second Conference on the teaching of general practice (the

Leeuwenhorst Conference)[6] which complemented those of *The Future General Practitioner* and agreed with the educational objectives for child health, psychiatry and geriatrics published jointly with the British Paediatric Association, the Royal College of Psychiatrists and the British Geriatrics Society[7]. The basis of the examination therefore became increasingly well defined and the Panel was required to ensure adequate assessment of a wide diversity of educational objectives. Although this proved to be possible only on the basis of sampling (the educational objectives for child health alone would have required a special examination), the mixture of techniques and a judicious selection of topics allowed a considerable number of objectives to be assessed.

In each examination, the 90-question multiple-choice paper (MCQ) assessed factual knowledge over the full range of general practice, the modified essay question (MEQ) the candidates' problem-solving ability in one or more clinical areas, and the traditional essay question (TEQ) his skill in marshalling facts and arguments in the areas of human behaviour, health-care organization, and clinical practice. The oral examinations reinforced the papers and provided the opportunity for more personal evaluation of the candidates' approach to general practice and, in particular, their methods of thought in problem-solving and the management of hypothetical clinical situations.

Setting and Marking Examinations

Each of the techniques used in the examination was developed independently. Multiple-choice questions were constructed by individual examiners, edited by two coordinators and validated by a small experienced group within the panel. The modified essay questions were constructed by a small group of examiners, edited by a larger group and validated by being answered by all panel members. A marking schedule was developed and marks were allocated to each section by the group. In a similar way the traditional-essay questions were constructed by small groups who were also responsible for producing the outline answer for each. In turn, this was submitted to a larger group for comment. As a result of these procedures and through work at the Examiners' Conferences, all examiners were involved in the construction of each written paper, and assumed responsibility for its content and validity.

Marking in the case of the multiple-choice question paper was by computer. As well as providing analyses of candidate performance, the programme evaluated the discriminating ability of each question. Poor discriminators were identified and questions which, despite preliminary vetting, were shown to be unsatisfactory, were eliminated from the calculation of the mark.

While the computer could mark MCQs, the marking of the essays had to be undertaken by examiners. Each TEQ and each page of the MEQ was assessed independently by two examiners and any significant discrepancy was considered by a third. Each candidate's Part I mark was therefore the product of the work of at least 30 examiners – six who set the MCQ paper, six who marked the TEQ paper, and 20 who marked the MEQ paper.

In the early days of the examination the calculations at this stage were completed by hand. As the number of candidates and of examiners increased, this became difficult and the Computing Laboratory in the University of Newcastle upon Tyne developed a programme which carried out the mathematical tasks and also provided analyses of candidate and examiner performance which allowed discrepancies to be rapidly identified and reliability assessed.

Candidates whose performance in the written papers was deemed to be satisfactory were invited to attend the oral examination six weeks later. In the interim they had completed and sent to the College a Log Diary describing the practice in which they worked and listing 50 consecutive patients. This Log Diary formed the basis of the first oral examination in which the candidate could be examined in relation to his own practice and to his own patients. The second oral was more loosely structured and was based upon clinical and other problems produced by the examiner. Each of the orals lasted approximately 30 minutes and was conducted by two examiners, often in the presence of a third acting as an observer. The examiners were not aware of the candidate's marks on the written paper; and only when the final mark had been calculated did the four examiners come together to confer about any candidate whose mark placed him or her near the borderline. The important role which the oral examination played was recognized too and, for this reason, consistency of standards was of continuing concern to the panel. The answers to MCQs were determined by reference to standard works and recent publications. Ideal answers to the MEQs and TEQs were established by consensus within the panel. Standards of the oral examination were essentially the responsibility of individual pairs of examiners and the quartets of examiners who discussed the border-line candidate. Examiners who acted as observers were able both to learn and to criticize constructively. Continued analysis during the examination and refinement of the aims and techniques of the oral remained high priorities.

Clinical Competence

The absence of a clinical component in the examination then had frequently been a cause for comment. Many clinical competences could be assessed realistically during a conventional oral examination, and many more clinical situations could be covered hypothetically without the presence of patients. A variety of experimental techniques, however, were being developed to increase the validity of the clinical components of the examination and allow competence in this field to be assessed more directly.

Results

On the conclusion of the oral examination the results of the examination were published. Both successful and unsuccessful candidates were offered information about their marks in each of the components of the examination. These might then become the subject of congratulation or counselling.

Although the examination was not without its critics, many candidates stated that it presented them with a fair and demanding test of knowledge and ability over a wide range of topics. A small number of existing members and fellows used the examination as a form of self-assessment; several took it and passed it twice! Their favourable comments encouraged the examiners in their belief that they had established a fair, reliable and relevant assessment of many of the competences of general practice.

Further Use of Data obtained at Examinations

Data from the earlier examinations only provided information about pass rates. As the number of candidates and the importance of the examination increased, it became obvious that more detailed analysis of the results was required to provide information for those involved in vocational training. In 1976 the application form for the examination was revised and candidates were invited to give much more detailed information. The computing laboratory in Newcastle once again provided the appropriate expert facility and the College was able to produce analyses which described and evaluated the internal processes of the examination and related these to the personal and professional characteristics of the candidate.

Recognition of our College's Diplomas

After the College had received its Royal Prefix in 1967 the General Medical Council and the Editor of *The Medical Directory* recognized the FRCGP and MRCGP diplomas.

Review

During the late 1960s and in the 1970s, the MRCGP examination (with the Court of Examiners chaired by P. S. Byrne) had developed and matured steadily and achieved the satisfactory and acceptable method of assessment which it has reached today.

The number of applicants for membership increased steadily, and soon the need for several centres was realized. It was decided that the written papers could be taken in Belfast, Cardiff, Edinburgh, Manchester and London. For the academic year 1977–78, 25 years after the foundation of the College, a total of 828 candidates went forward for the MRCGP examination.

This development of the examination was one of the outstanding, unsung success stories of our College's early life. It played a part in achieving what at one time appeared impossible – the development of an essential, but undefined, branch of medicine into one which through the use of contemporary clinical, educational and examination techniques could be taught, learnt and tested.

References

1. College of General Practitioners (1954). *Second Annual Report*. Appendix V. Criteria for Membership, 88–92
2. College of General Practitioners (1957). *Fifth Annual Report*. Report on Criteria for Continuing Membership, 34–40
3. Pickering, G. (1961). Examination in general practice. *Br. Med. J.,* **ii**, 1642
4. Royal College of General Practitioners (1969). Report of a conference on examination methods held on November 14 and 15 1968 at the Royal College of Physicians, London. *J. R. Coll. Gen. Practit.* **17**, 112–114
5. Royal College of General Practitioners (1972). *The Future General Practitioner. Learning and Teaching.* (London: British Medical Journal)
6. European Conference on the Teaching of General Practice (1976). The General Practitioner in Europe. *Med. Educ.,* **10**, 235–236
7. Royal College of General Practitioners (1978). *Some Aims for Training for General Practice.* Occasional Paper 6. (London: RCGP)

XI
THE COLLEGE AND RESEARCH

R. J. F. H. Pinsent and G. Ian Watson*

INTRODUCTION

The first and last in a series are said to be atypical. This can certainly be said of the beginning of the research activity for which the College became responsible. There were almost no precedents, little tradition of research existed, published work was minimal except from the pens of exceptional general practitioners of the calibre of Budd, Huxham, Jenner, Mackenzie and Pickles, who committed their own ideas to paper, producing original work of a highly individual and personal character.

There had been one attempt at coordinated research by general practitioners in the late nineteenth century when an experiment was made to collect opinions from doctors in practice on such questions as the possible infectivity of tuberculosis and the cause of syphilis. An international endeavour resulted in the collection of a large amount of information, the analysis of which proved impossible with the knowledge available to the practitioners of the day. The effort had been made, though, and the attempt was known to the members of the Steering Committee which, early in its work, accepted that research would be a proper outlet for the activity of any future College. While not something in which every doctor would be expected to engage, a particular kind of research, in the context of practice, seemed essential if progress made in other fields of medicine was to be equalled.

Two kinds of research suggested themselves, clinical and operational. Clinical research implied study of conditions met with in practice, and was in effect a kind of epidemiology differing from that of the infectious

---

* Ian Watson died on June 3 1979 just after he had completed his share of this chapter.

131

diseases. Experimental clinical research had little place in general practice, where situations could not be contrived and the terms of service of the National Health Service committed doctors to prescribe all proper and necessary treatment for their patients.

Much use of operational research had been made during World War II, of which all the members of the Steering Committee had had experience, when it was essential to find out how to do things effectively and economically, perhaps under difficult conditions. Of all kinds of medical practice general practice was most uneven in its conduct, and it appeared that practical steps to improve performance could only follow deliberate study of the many ways in which it was carried on. The Steering Committee decided that a Research Committee of Council, if set up, would encourage development along both lines.

Any account of the developments of the next 25 years must suffer from both omissions and summarization which may do less than justice to the work that was done and the people who did it. It is the story of amateur enthusiasm changed under the pressure of its own successes into a kind of professionalism which could only have originated in general practice.

For convenience of presentation the organizational needs will be described first, followed by an account of their application to clinical and observational research in general practice.

ORGANIZATION AND METHODS

The Research Committee of Council

The first meeting of the Research Committee of the Foundation Council was convened by R. J. F. H. Pinsent on March 29 1953, four months after the foundation of the College. The chosen site was Bath, equidistant from the homes of its furthest members, G. F. Abercrombie and J. H. Hunt in London, G. I. Watson in Surrey, D. G. French in Kidsgrove and R. M. S. McConaghey in Dartmouth.

The first and most encouraging response to the opening of a Research Register was discussed, as were the composition of the Research Advisory Panel, and plans for an investigation of the use of sulphonamides and antibiotics in the prevention of complications of measles which was tabled by Ian Watson. First steps towards a National Morbidity Survey were considered and the introduction of a *Newsletter* was decided upon to foster contact between members whose names were on the rapidly growing Research Register. In a quite remarkable way this meeting charted the course of future developments over the next decade.

Because members lived at a distance from one another much of the work had to be done by correspondence, and a method of postal discussion with consolidation and recirculation of comments of members was introduced. This proved of value when the membership of the Committee increased, and saved much travelling. The first matters discussed were those of principle, evaluating needs and means of carrying out work of an acceptably high standard. Four kinds of interested practitioner were recognized – those wishing to work alone, perhaps towards an MD thesis, those prepared to work with others in an interest group, those willing to collect information on behalf of centrally directed studies, and doctors willing to devise and develop research methods for general use, testing these in their own practices.

Research Committees of Faculties

Methods were needed to establish the nature, kind and amount of diseases met with and managed in general practice, and to carry out their proper investigation. To do these things it was necessary to create some kind of ordered framework within which enthusiastic members of a profession not noted for its singlemindedness could work usefully together. Advantage was taken of the faculty structure decided upon by Council, and as a first step Research members were appointed to faculty Research Committees which acted as local foci of interest near the homes of doctors in practice. The Research Committee of Council appreciated the dangers which might arise from overcentralization. By decentralization not only were local problems identified, but new workers were brought to light, some of whom attended the regular meetings of the Research Committee of Council as these began to assume a more or less regular pattern.

The need for research at practice level was also stressed by conferences to which faculty research representatives were invited. Some faculties were, from the start, more active in research than others, for reasons which were partly concerned with personalities. Where an exceptionally enthusiastic and able research worker stimulated local studies good progress was made, though this inevitably slowed when his abilities, as frequently happened, led to his co-option to the Research Committee of Council. The faculty structure encouraged research by groups of doctors in addition to work originated by the Research Committee of Council itself, but a pattern evolved in which proposals for faculty studies were often referred to the central Committee as much for advice as for approval. Though very conscious of its inexperience, the Research Committee of Council was forced to accept an advisory function.

None of the members of the early Faculty Research Committees had received formal training in the research field, all were in active practice and thus familiar with its circumstances. The committee usually accepted advice. The Research Support Unit was set up, under the wing of the Research Committee of Scottish Council and J. D. E. Knox in the University of Dundee. Whereas this was largely a College research unit, the universities themselves soon followed, on both sides of the border, setting up projects with the support and help of the faculty of the College in which the medical school was situated.

Research Methods

It had been hoped that existing research methods could be adapted for use in practice, but it soon became clear that this was not so. The pace of practice, and the opportunities it provided for the making of a few observations at many consultations, contrasted with hospital practice in which many observations could be made on a relatively few patients. One asset on which we could call, however, was the burgeoning science of statistics which was beginning to gain respectability in the eyes of the medical profession. It was becoming possible to handle, even by manual means, very large amounts of data. In this the Research Committee of Council was particularly fortunate. It had, however, to face the problems associated with the collection of material for statistical analysis. Much experience was gained in the planning and conduct of the first National Morbidity Survey, which will be described later with other methods of general-practitioner research.

The Use of Statistical Methods

Soon after the establishment of the Epidemic Observation Unit in the South, activity accelerated in the Midlands where, by good fortune, Professor Lancelot Hogben and Dr Kenneth Cross of the Department of Medical Statistics in the University of Birmingham were interested in the demography of disease, and the stage was set for work on new ways of collecting and preparing statistically-useful material from the tremendous volume of general practice. It had also to be shown that the statistical method could be applied to the therapeutic research in practice as well as operational research, in both of which Hogben had had wartime experience. The College has had no better guide to the reduction of the complex issues of practice to mathematical terms. Both Hogben and Cross were recruited to the Research Advisory Panel.

Methods of Recording

To enable practice research data to be properly analysed its collection must be carried out within a framework determined by statistical considerations. The 'E' Book, and subsequently the Diagnostic Index, were designed with this in mind.

The 'E' Book and the Diagnostic Index

The ledger which came to be called the 'E' Book[1], after its originator T. S. Eimerl, was one in which banks of overlapping data sheets were carried in the pocket. In its original form the identities of patients sharing a common condition were entered on the sheet allocated to that condition. The Research Committee developed the principle in two main ways. First, it allocated a diagnostic rubric and code number to each looseleaf sheet, and had it printed on the cards which separated sets of sheets. Second, it adjusted the layout of the data sheets themselves so that information entered could be directly, and easily, converted to punch-cards for mechanical handling and analysis. In its developed form the 'E' Book became the Diagnostic Index and as such was, and is, widely used at home and overseas. It had solved the problem, posed by the first National Morbidity Survey, that data should be coded at practice headquarters.

Though doctors introducing the diagnostic index to their practices normally made the entries themselves between consultations, at least to begin with, it was always intended that maintaining the index should be a secretarial task. Thus was conceived the idea of the research secretary in a partnership practice who would maintain research documentation for the whole practice and be involved in whatever special studies were carried out. It was to be her task too to make periodic returns to the central unit set up by the Research Committee where a data-bank was forming, capable of use in many different ways.

Age–Sex Register

Attention was paid, also, to a further variable – that practices varied in their composition. To effect proper comparisons between practices it was necessary to express figures as percentages and this could not be done without some kind of register. The practice stock of medical record envelopes, filed in drawers, or on shelves, constituted a register of a kind, but it did not meet the need. The first Age–Sex Registers were therfore redesigned so that their contents could be used as punch-cards for computer input.

The 'S' Card

The third dimension which called for the introduction of new methods was that of the patient himself and his consecutive illnesses from infancy onwards. This could not readily be discovered from a diagnostic index, and a prototype individual summary card proposed by James Scott of Keele was developed by the Research Committee in the same way as the data sheet in the diagnostic index[2]. This record was kept with patients' documents.

Scott's work marked the beginning of a new stage – the commitment to research of the University Departments of General Practice which were to come.

The Research Register

At first the work of building up a Research Register, classifying doctors who volunteered because of interests or opportunities in their practices, was done in the homes of those involved. As the work intensified it was shared. C. A. H. Watts and Elizabeth Watts became the first Registrars to the Research Committee, with responsibility for maintaining a register which at one time included nearly 400 doctors' names.

The Research Newsletter

To bring information to the notice of members on the Research Register some means of communication was necessary, and the Research *Newsletter,* decided upon at the first meeting of the Research Committee of Council, first appeared in the autumn of 1953. This *Newsletter*, and subsequent ones, were published by the editor of *The Practitioner* and thus reached a far wider audience. When this *Newsletter* was developed into the *Journal* of the College a more restricted means of communication was still necessary. The need was met by an informal circular titled *Between Ourselves*. This served for several years as a clearing house for ideas particularly relating to the new methods of research which were being explored.

The Records and Statistical Unit

It became clear that there were limits to the output of spare-time practitioner workers, unless they had secretarial help. From this small beginning stemmed the Records and Statistical Unit of the College, with the full support of the Birmingham Regional Hospital Board, which also offered the unit office accommodation. The unit began to explore not only the quantification of doctors' work on the morbidity which he encountered, but also other and more fundamental issues such as the ethics of research in practice, confidentiality of data, the conduct of therapeutic trials and the important matter of the future finance of research in general practice. It was set up in Birmingham. As its responsibilities increased it was later reconstituted as the Birmingham Research Unit and Donald L. Crombie became its director. It was from Birmingham that the planning of the first National Morbidity Survey began in 1954. This is described below (page 141).

The reports of the first National Morbidity Survey[3] were widely used as a new baseline for epidemiological studies. Among the other lessons learned was that, given the right methods and good central organization, doctors in general practice could become field observers achieving a good standard of accuracy and consistency throughout prolonged studies. This was appreciated by the Research Committee and it was the task of the unit in Birmingham to work out methods of collection of data from general practice and to provide a central focus for the initiation and conduct of other studies. Many of its difficulties arose from the lack of definitions for the conditions met within general practice. An urgent necessity was a classification of disease appropriate to practice circumstances.

The unit's first classification was arranged hierarchically at four levels. This was soon replaced by a short list from the International Classification of Diseases and Causes of Death (ICD).

It was through involvement with other users of general-practice classifications, particularly in Canada, Australia and the United States, that the opportunity to develop the College Classification of Diagnoses into a truly international one first arose. It had been realized that more than diagnoses required to be classified and from intensive discussions under a Canadian chairman a new classification was evolved, the International Classification of Health Problems in Primary Care (ICHPPC)[4]. This classification was accepted by the World Organization of National Colleges and Academies of General Practice (WONCA) in 1974 and gradually superseded the original College Classification in the Diagnostic Indexes and Morbidity Indexes in the world.

Terms and Definitions

A glossary of terms and definitions used in research in general practice had been produced in Birmingham. The second edition[5] of this incorporated some definitions in current use overseas; but this, too, was clearly capable of further development, and the task was taken up by WONCA. The reconciliation of different concepts of diagnoses as well as diagnostic terminologies proved a formidable challenge to the new WONCA committee entrusted with the task. Countries throughout the world are represented on this committee.

The Research Advisory Service

With the wide awakening of interest in research, the Research Committee was continually called upon for advice and help not only by practising doctors but also by people working in other fields of medicine and science. Meeting these needs required time and resources and these were made available to a specially constituted Research Advisory Service. R. J. F. H. Pinsent was appointed Research Adviser.

The operation of the practice in which he worked, and the activities of the Research Unit itself, provided the necessary resources and teaching material. Visitors to the Research Unit were numerous, for discussions on the setting up of studies or the analysis of practice material. Those wishing to see the standardized procedures of research documentation in use went first to the Birchfield Study Practice where the staff who took the active part in handling research data were available to describe their work. When the decision was made to base the second National Morbidity Survey on diagnostic indexes and age–sex registers, preliminary planning and teaching went on at both places.

The building of new premises for D. L. Crombie's practice provided the opportunity to house the Research Unit, of which he was director. Lordswood House, in Harborne, became the first purpose-built research centre for general practice. It accommodated the Research Adviser and received problems which were referred from College headquarters in London and those which came from general practitioners direct. The new building was opened in 1973, its staff including a business manager with secretarial support and statistics clerks to handle the ever-increasing amount of work. The unit became the supply centre for special documents for use in general-practice research.

Co-operation with the Office of Population Censuses and Surveys

The second National Morbidity Survey[6] was undertaken by the College and the Office of Population Censuses and Surveys into which the General Register Office had by then metamorphosed. It was financed by the DHSS which covered support costs at the centre and in the practices taking part. Confidentiality of recorded data had become an issue and this was overcome by arranging for age–sex cards identifying patients to be handled separately from morbidity data on diagnostic index sheets. The two were subsequently matched in the impersonal neutrality of the OPCS computers. The College Classification was somewhat altered and improved for use in the survey. Practices were enrolled, procedures explained at regional meetings, and data collection began in 1971. In this survey about the same number of doctors took part as in the first survey, but in fewer practices because, since then, there had been a strong trend, countrywide, towards group and partnership practices.

Council Representation

To begin with, the work of the Research Committee was shared among its members, who developed postal consideration of problems to a high degree. The formation of Research Units, however, concentrated experience and activity into fewer hands. This was recognized by the creation of the Research Division of the College, the executive of which consisted of the Directors of the Research Units, together with certain co-options. This streamlining of what had become a cumbersome committee was further evidence of the achievement of a new level of maturity.

CLINICAL AND OBSERVATIONAL RESEARCH IN GENERAL PRACTICE

The Epidemic Observation Unit

In the epidemiological field, statutory notification systems already existed for a number of serious infectious diseases. One of the first tasks undertaken by the Epidemic Observation Unit was to extend this work, introducing a system of voluntary notification of the occurrence of statutory non-notifiable epidemics such as Bornholm disease[7] and Epidemic Winter Vomiting[8]

William Pickles had already investigated the development and spread of infective hepatitis, which was not notifiable at that time. His observations had already modified the textbooks.

The Epidemic Observation Unit was set up in Surrey by G. I. Watson, who had gone into practice there soon after the war, and was a member of the Research Committee of the Foundation Council.

The Public Health Laboratory Service, with headquarters at Colindale, was a result of the wartime organization there, and discussions revealed the need for information about epidemic diseases which were not statutorily notifiable. Ian Watson set himself to work out methods whereby symptom-patterns observed in general practice were circulated to members on the research register who were alerted to the possibility of finding them in their own practices also. In this way Bornholm disease, Epidemic Winter Vomiting and various outbreaks of 'influenza' were studied, as were clinical presentations often involving pyrexia and rashes. These might have had no name and were identified by their place of origin, such as 'Shere fever' from the village of Shere in Ian Watson's practice, or by a compound code-number including the initial of the reporting doctor, that of the place, and the year. KL57 was a condition reported to the Epidemic Observation Unit by F. E. B. Kelly of Leicester in 1957.

The first concern of the Epidemic Observation Unit was the study of the movement of infections through the country, epidemiology of the type which Pickles had introduced into general practice. Ian Watson added a new dimension – the study of the movement of infectious illness within the family – using serological titre changes as an indicator. Public Health Laboratory Service laboratories throughout the country collaborated, and combined studies of the movement of virologically confirmed influenza began. On the national scale, map plots were made relating the observed morbidity to the geographical environment. The work of the Epidemic Observation Unit and the Records and Statistical Unit was complementary, each supported the other.

With the retirement from the Epidemic Observation Unit of G. I. Watson the opportunity was taken to divide its functions between a reconstituted Epidemic Observation Unit under Paul Grob, based at Addlestone and within the University of Surrey. The inclination of this unit was toward the relationship of disease to its environment; and a new unit under W. O. Williams was set up in Swansea with interests more along traditional epidemiological lines. It was to develop as a centre for the study of the spread of disease nationally and through communities. Interest in other aspects of the relationship between the patterns of illness in a given place and the characteristics of the local environment had concerned the Research Committee for some time.

Therapeutic Trials

It had been hoped that therapeutic trials of new medicines could be carried out in practice as they were in hospitals; but it was soon found that to do so would require doctors to break the terms of their contract under the National Health Service. The legal implications were explored and a decision made that certain kinds of study could be legitimately suggested by the College but not necessarily conducted by it.

The First National Morbidity Survey

Partly through the *Research Newsletter* and partly by direct contact, a group of doctors was created to seek to achieve a more accurate picture of the distribution of morbidity – the pattern of illness in England and Wales. Planning and teaching had hitherto been based on mortality – the legacy of the legislation on the notification of births, marriages and deaths, passed at the turn of the century. Lethal disease was, generally speaking, disease requiring hospital care and consequently assumed a disproportionate importance in the eyes of medical students who were taught there. The load of self-limiting disease had never been assessed except on a limited scale by E. M. Backett of the London School of Hygiene and by W. P. D. Logan of the General Register Office. There was a real need for a National Morbidity Survey, something which could only be carried out with the help of doctors in the field – those in general practice. The setting-up of a survey of this kind was a logical responsibility for the Research Committee of Council. A system of recording had to be devised from fundamentals, using the episode of illness as the denominator. Diagnoses were to be recorded by the doctors at the time of consultation. The age–sex distribution of the practice populations was to be based on censuses held in the practices during the survey year, together with details of occupation.

The enrolment of the practices was effected through the Research Register and a pilot study of the methods to be used was carried out in each. Modifications and adjustments were made and the main survey began in 1955. All episodes of illness occurring in the practices during one year were recorded, including those requiring no treatment beyond that which the doctor could provide as well as those needing hospital care. During the survey year the practices were visited by members of the staff of the General Register Office to clarify any difficulties in record-keeping which may have arisen, and to ensure comparability as far as was possible. Recording information of this kind was a new experience for doctors and their staffs. Those organizing the study and those who took part in it learned many lessons.

The first of these was that, where doctors recorded diagnoses in their own words, these had to be coded centrally before statistical analysis was possible, and the coding of the output of 171 doctors in 106 practices during the survey year was a mammoth undertaking. Sixteen coding clerks were employed for six months converting diagnoses into terms compatible with the *International Classification of Diseases and Causes of Death*. At the same time occupations were coded using standard General Register Office (GRO) procedures, as were the social classes of patients, using the five-point classification previously adopted by the General Register Office.

141

It had been decided that the analysis of the accumulated information would be presented in three reports in the appropriate series published by Her Majesty's Stationery Office (HMSO)[3]. The first volume contained the statistical material following an account of the planning and methods used. The second related the tabulated materials to the occupations of those who had been ill, and the third was a largely narrative interpretation of the figures. This third volume, which appeared in 1962, broke new ground, for it was written and edited by some of the general practitioners who had taken part in the study itself instead of by members of the Civil Service.

Research Projects by General Practitioners

The Oral Contraception Study

The Steering Committee had realized that it should be the responsibility of the College to study the application of advances in medical knowledge to the work and conduct of general practice. At a meeting of the Research Committee of Council in 1965, E. V. Kuenssberg proposed an investigation into the possible effects of oral contraception on women who adopted this form of family planning. Preliminary discussions in Birmingham indicated that the scale on which the study would have to be mounted justified the creation of a separate Research Unit and this was set up under Clifford Kay in Manchester. The genesis and development of the project merits consideration in some detail as it exemplified the principles which lie behind the establishment of any major study. The Research Committee of Council was by now finding its feet in the world of research and had the beginnings of a real understanding of what was needed.

The first stage was recognition of the existence of a problem which could best be examined in general practice. Certainly oral contraception presented such a problem. Its long-term consequences were then unknown, while its immediate effectiveness guaranteed its use by large numbers of women. Consultation with others, including the Family Planning Association and the pharmaceutical manufacturing houses, confirmed that there was indeed a problem here. Next, the right man had to be found with the enthusiasm and ability to plan the study and carry it through. Following its now customary procedure the Research Committee appointed Clifford Kay as 'Recorder' of the project, and supported him with a small planning team of members of the committee, with others.

An appropriate method had to be devised, in this instance involving a large number of doctors. The documentation and procedure had to work under all circumstances of practice, and pilot trials were carried out before enrolment of observers could begin. The observers came from all parts of the country, and local meetings attended by the Recorder and members of the planning team were arranged to explain the study. Although those who took part in the collection of information were volunteers, some small recompense to cover expenses was met from the central grant, partly from the Medical Research Council, partly from the pharmaceutical manufacturers, with a contribution from the Research Foundation of the College. This study[9] established the Manchester Research Unit of the College as a unit capable of handling very large amounts of data from a very large number of doctors. The multi-observer study in which the number of observers exceeds 1000 was shown to be practicable and sound in the only field in which it could be undertaken – general medical practice.

Environment and Disease

As far back as 1960 a report[10] by E. V. Allen-Price had suggested that cancer of the stomach occurred in abnormal clusters in West Devon and East Cornwall, and by 1963 the Research Committee's data collection methods were advanced enough for a study to be set up to determine whether other disturbances of the pattern of morbidity could be detected in the Tamar Valley which divides Devon from Cornwall. Practices in the area, which included that from which Allen-Price had reported, were invited to maintain diagnostic indexes. They did so for a year and a half, covering a population of approximately 20 000. Data from this source were compared with similar data from practices far away from the specified locality. Comparisons showed abnormal prevalence of certain other conditions in the Tamar Valley, within the limits set by the study. The results suggested that some factor might be operating in the area to disturb the morbidity pattern.

Consideration of various possibilities led to the conclusion that the known abnormal mineralization of the Tamar Valley, from natural sources and the results of nineteenth century mining, might be relevant. A series of investigations was begun by non-medical scientists to determine the extent of which, if any, trace elements from the environment entered the food chain which ended in the inhabitants of the locality. The first lettuce samples from the area were analysed in the laboratories of Professor H. V. Warren of the Department of Geological Sciences in the University of British Columbia. Later, other workers including Dr Brian Davies (of the University of Wales at Aberystwyth) and Professor C. Webb (of Imperial College, London) became involved in local environmental studies.

As interest in environmentally related disease grew, two annual conferences – 'Airs, Waters and Places'[11] – were held at College headquarters. These were invitation conferences with distinguished speakers from this country and North America. Wide-ranging discussions took place; each conference concluded that there was no better place for the study of disease than in the environment in which it occurs. It was emphasized that data from general practice can demonstrate abnormalities of distribution of disease where these cannot otherwise be recognized, and lead to investigations by others to prove or disprove causal relationships. In these activities the Research Committee of Council was demonstrating its maturity without being aware that it was doing so, for the influence of research in general practice was now extending beyond the discipline of medicine into wider fields of science. The links established between the Research Committee and the earth scientists are now strong, and will strengthen further.

Genetically Determined Diseases

The international expansion of research in general practice will undoubtedly encourage research into genetically determined diseases and those conditions which may be found to be precipitated by a combination of both. That planned international studies can be carried out was shown by the College's work comparing morbidity patterns in populations of different ancestral origin in Newfoundland, South-west England and Southern Ireland. A beginning had been made in exploring a dimension of international epidemiology which can be advanced in no better context than general practice.

The European General Practice Research Unit

Diagnostic Indexes had been sent to doctors in practice in countries throughout and beyond the English-speaking world. The Research Committee of Council found itself having to think internationally long before any question of entry into the European Community arose.

In Holland the Diagnostic Index had been used as part of the data-collection system in the first National Morbidity Survey to be carried out in that country.

Many visitors to the College and to the Birmingham Unit were from overseas, and both the director and research adviser were invited to visit practice centres and developing research units overseas. In particular, they became involved in the work of the Research Committee of the World Organization of National Colleges and Academies of General Practice.

A logical consequence was the setting up of the *European General*

Practice Research Unit under the chairmanship of E. V. Kuenssberg. Those concerned were surprised to find how little difficulty language presented, and how readily methods worked out in the United Kingdom could be picked up and used in other countries. A mutual exchange of methods and ideas began, and is continuing fruitfully.

THE RESEARCH FOUNDATION, EDUCATION FOUNDATION AND SCIENTIFIC FOUNDATION

Ekke V. Kuenssberg

Development of research in general practice had shown the need for improvisation to overcome the lack of formal funding. For some years all research organized for, and carried out in general practice was done at the expense of the doctors who took part. Gradually funding of studies became easier following a proposal by R. M. S. McConaghey that the College should itself set aside some of its resources and create a *Research Foundation*. Money for this purpose was administered separately from other College funds by a Board of Trustees. Over the years this Foundation assisted in the planning and pilot-testing of many projects later supported from other sources on a larger scale. Many more smaller studies were completely financed, and numerous travel grants were awarded to enable doctors to attend and speak at conferences overseas. The latter activity carried an educational element and Council decided that the funds set aside for research should be continued with those earmarked for the support of education for general practice. From the merger of trusts the Scientific Foundation of the College came into being to serve similar functions at a lower administrative cost.

The development of this Scientific Foundation has its separate existence within the College organization, basically to avoid rivalry between the College's housekeeping finance and what had been collected through various appeals and donations, bequests and gifts for such special purposes as research, prizes or other purely academic ventures.

Under the chairmanship of W. J. H. (Jack) Lord, a Planning Committee of the Research Committee of Council in 1959 made recommendations that were based on the realization and fact-finding that general-practice research and teaching were inadequately financed, particularly during the stage of early development. After taking stock of the activities of other grant-giving bodies, it was recommended to Council that the College should set up its own Research Trust, financed from its own Appeal monies. (It might well have declared the Research Committee of Council the appropriate Trustee or Board to administer such a fund; but as the researchers

145

represented on the Research Committee were possibly the first, and most likely, applicants for such support, it was decided to have a Board of Trustees, on which some eminent persons outside the College would be invited to serve alongside Council-appointed members.)

In 1960 the Research Foundation was set up. Sir Harry Jephcott and Lord Cohen of Birkenhead played important parts in the planning committee (chaired by E. V. Kuenssberg). Sir Harry became the first chairman, in May 1961, when the standing committee handed over to the fully constituted Foundation, all legal steps having been taken. Three years later the *Education Foundation* (first chairman Sir Max (later Lord) Rosenheim) followed the same pattern, to finance educational ventures.

The two Foundations, through their respective Boards, soon developed considerable expertise and experience on what needed their support, and what could be presented to a more amply endowed grant-giving body. The best example was the pre-pilot and pilot surveys necessary before we could convince the Medical Research Council of the soundness of our oral contraception study, requiring £3000 over two years from the Foundation.

The presence of outstanding scientists and educationalists on these Foundations was a considerable tribute to the College's work and for what it stood.

It became obvious that administrative costs could be halved, and Trust Funds more purposefully allocated, when the two Foundations joined forces, and became renamed *The Scientific Foundation* (AGM, 1976) under the vigorous and constructive chairmanship of Sir George Godber, who had just laid down the burden of Chief Medical Officer to the Department of Health and Social Security.

References

1. Eimerl, T. S. (1960, 1961). Organized curiosity. *J. Coll. Gen. Practit.,* **3**, 246–252; **4**, 628–631
2. Royal College of General Practitioners (1972). The analysis of summarized data using 'S' cards. Research Unit. *J. R. Coll. Gen. Practit.,* **22**, 377–381
3. General Register Office (1958–1962). *Morbidity Statistics from General Practice.* (London: HMSO)
4. World Organization of National Colleges, Academies and Academic Associations of General Practitioners (1979). *ICHPPC-Z.* (Oxford: OUP)
5. Royal College of General Practitioners (1973). A general-practice glossary. 2nd edn. *J. R. Coll. Gen. Practit.,* **23**, Suppl. 3
6. Royal College of General Practitioners, Office of Population Censuses and Surveys and Department of Health and Social Security (1974). *Morbidity Statistics from General Practice.* Second National Study 1970–71. (London: HMSO)
7. College of General Practitioners (1957). Bornholm disease 1956. *Research Newsletter,* **NS 4**, 155–121

8. College of General Practitioners (1955). Epidemic winter vomiting. *Research Newsletter, NS* **2,** 96–98

9. Royal College of General Practitioners (1974). *Oral Contraceptives and Health.* An interim report from the Oral Contraception Study. (Tunbridge Wells: Pitman)

10. Allen-Price, E. D. (1960). Uneven distribution of cancer in West Devon. *Lancet,* **i,** 1235–1238

11. Royal College of General Practitioners (1971). Airs, waters and places. *J. R. Coll. Gen. Practit.,* **21,** 682–686

147

XII
PRACTICE ORGANIZATION, EQUIPMENT AND PREMISES

George S. Adams and Michael Drury

From the earliest days of the College the founding members believed that organization and management should be encouraged. Prior to the College's foundation, general practice was sometimes considered a 'cottage industry' and the Collings Report, *A Survey of General Practice*[1], of 1950 gave much support to that premise, laying emphasis on the poor conditions under which some general practitioners worked. The challenge of improving this state of affairs was taken up by the Nuffield Provincial Hospitals Trust who sponsored a study in depth of general practice by Stephen Taylor (later Lord Taylor).

His investigations were undertaken at the same time as the first members were laying foundations for a College for general practitioners and the publication *Good General Practice*[2] in 1954 by Dr Taylor gave a balanced and helpful view of the problem.

From its earliest days the College Council considered how to interest members and associates in the study of practice organization. In 1953 the Council set up an Equipment and Premises Committee, with a panel of architects instructed and knowledgeable in the solution of the problems. It was hoped that in time one or more local architects would be co-opted to each Faculty Board.

In 1953 the establishment of an 'Institute of General Practice' was being discussed. This was to concentrate on practice organization by the College with other interested groups, and its purpose was stated to be:

To give instruction in various techniques, types and use of equipment, organisation of work and premises and the training of secretaries and technical assistants. In addition, advice on

149

architectural details for those planning alteration and extension of premises, or the development of a group practice or health centre, would be available; all this being supported by plans and photographs of work already carried out ...

The study of this project bore no fruit, for the College had already preempted these objectives.

EARLY COLLEGE SURVEY

Practice organization was soon being pursued by the regional faculties. The South-East Scotland faculty (under the chairmanship of E. V. Kuenssberg) carried out a survey of the equipment, buildings and administration requirements of their members which was published in 1956 as an *Index of Equipment with Photographs and Plans of General Practitioners' Surgeries*. In 1956 the Northern Home Counties faculty made visits to practices in Ashford, Southall and Thaxted to study the problem within the practice setting. The South London faculty set up an Equipment and Premises Subcommittee of its Postgraduate Education Committee. Meanwhile, the Postgraduate Education Committee of Council had considered the problem and made suggestions in its annual report to Council in 1956 as follows:

> *The Professional Accommodation and Equipment of Family Doctors and those intending to enter general practice.*
> It has been suggested that these aspects of the work of a faculty may appropriately be considered and directed at present by an Equipment and Premises Subcommittee of the Postgraduate Education Committee of the Faculty Board. They are closely bound up with the requirements of those about to enter general practice, and with the problems involved in helping family doctors to keep up-to-date. One of the functions of the College will be to act as a centre for information for young practitioners on their needs in general practice, on methods of record keeping, on new methods for diagnosis or treatment, and on the equipment needed for these.... By this means they will choose their equipment and establish themselves in general practice more easily and more quickly than they can at present.

Such a subcommittee would be concerned with:

(1) Questions connected with general practitioners' premises – waiting rooms, dispensaries, consulting room etc.

(2) The administrative problems and record systems of family doctors, including details of the charts (temperature, diabetic, intake and output, menstruation etc) and diet sheets, needed by family doctors to make sure that these were the best for their use.

(3) The apparatus used by family doctors.

PRACTICE EQUIPMENT AND PREMISES COMMITTEE

During 1956 the Council decided that the subject of the accommodation and equipment of general practitioners was of sufficient importance to merit a separate committee of Council. This was given the title of The Practice Equipment and Premises Committee and commenced work in 1957 with John Sanctuary as Chairman, George Adams as honorary secretary, and J. Fry, I.M. Hunter, D. Scott Napier, G. Swift, G. Little, J.G. Ollerenshaw, S. Taylor and P. Walford.

The first committee was inexperienced and unsure of how to fulfil its function for, apart from Stephen Taylor's *Good General Practice,* there was no corpus of knowledge to fall back on. It was decided to divide practice descriptions into six parts:

(1) The practice and its organization.
(2) Accommodation and how it was used.
(3) Finance.
(4) Architect's plans.
(5) Photographs.
(6) Comments and criticisms.

Each faculty was then asked to obtain as many planned descriptions as possible. The response was excellent, and by 1959 there was at headquarters a collection of practice descriptions available for anyone to study. Mr C. Verity, of Foster Wheeler Ltd, most generously offered to duplicate these so that if a doctor made an enquiry about practice organization we could respond by loaning him relevant descriptions of similar practices. Under Mrs Eileen Phillips, secretary to the Committee, this scheme developed.

A Display Room

So that greater use could be made of the material which this committee was collecting, a room was made available at College headquarters, then at 41 Cadogan Gardens. The committee not only had practice descriptions on display and available for perusal but also three display cabinets wherein to mount static demonstrations. The first three subjects chosen were:

(1) A general practitioner's house visiting case accompanied by a selection of basic items that should be carried in it.
(2) A midwifery case similarly equipped.
(3) A display of more sophisticated equipment – electrocardiogram, sigmoidoscope and a cautery set.

Allen and Hanbury Ltd most generously provided the showcases and the equipment on show.

This naturally led the committee to a study of the ideal bag for a doctor. It was found that one was not sufficient and that there should be three: one for normal visiting, one for emergencies and one for midwifery. A second investigation that resulted from this project was the study of the contents of these bags. When decided, printed and on display, the list of contents gave rise to a great deal of discussion amongst the visitors and many useful comments were made.

Comment System

From the early days of the committee requests for advice, plans, organization, financial and legal matters affecting practices, and for the names of architects, began to flow in – at first a trickle but soon a flood. Once again we had very little published work to guide us, but the Research Committee circulated enquiries for consideration and comment. This became known as the 'Consolidated Comment System'. Replies were consolidated and forwarded to the individual who had requested advice. Some of the requests for information were outside the knowledge of the members of the committee – usually on finance or legal matters. In these cases advice was taken from a friendly accountant or lawyer who gave his service free. Both the chairman and the honorary secretary had worked with an experienced architect, Mr Brian Peake, when developing their own practice premises, and whenever a problem arose he gave valuable help. In the same way most competent and sound advice on financial matters was given by Mr. B. Ducker without payment. The Committee had agreed that its service should be on a voluntary basis. Behind this decision was the thought that many other doctors would be unwilling to make requests if it was not a free service. This proved correct, as the principle was tested at a later date by another organization who found that enquiries dropped dramatically upon the introduction of a fee for services.

Record Cards

Much time was spent by the committee discussing the design of a *Summary Card* which carried details of the patient's serious illnesses, hereditary tendencies, immunization status and other matters. Nearly 53 000 of these were distributed in 1960. Later the committee designed an *Obstetric Card* which proved very popular and was the forerunner of the antenatal co-operation card.

The Council referred several issues to the Committee in 1958 – the draft antenatal co-operation card discussed with the Ministry of Health, a standard card on drug information (the forerunner of the data card) and the needs of the library.

Advisory Service on Premises and their Organization

Knowledge was accumulated and enquiries kept flowing. By 1961 the Committee had evolved a General Practice Advisory Service on Premises and their Organization. The figures revealed in the report to Council for that year of the number of doctors given advice in the year ended May 31 1961 were:

Plans of premises 33, Heating 10, Flooring 10, Lighting 7, Equipment 7, Records 7, Furniture 6, Appointments Systems 6, Call Systems 3, Sterilization Equipment 3, Loans 3, Soundproofing 2, Miscellaneous 3.

During the same year complete sets of the Practice Descriptions were placed in Scotland and Ireland. The Scottish Council established a Practice Equipment and Premises Room in Edinburgh with these. Those in Ireland were in the care of Dr Elizabeth Doherty in Dublin. For the first time demonstrations were mounted in the Practice Equipment and Premises Room. Dr M. Curwen of Margate, Kent, and Miss Bearup of the Royal Surrey County Hospital set up *Simple Aids for the Physically Handicapped in the Home* which stimulated much interest.

PRACTICE ORGANIZATION COMMITTEE

The advisory service began to attact a great deal of attention outside the College among general practitioners who were not College members. The committee decided that no one should be refused advice and, as its role expanded, it was thought the committee was inappropriately named. In

1961 Council accepted the recommendation that the committee should be renamed "The Practice Organization Committee". In addition, the Group Practice Loan Committee of the Ministry of Health asked the College to appoint an observer.

The secretary of the Practice Organization Committee began to make visits to practices to discuss practitioners' problems with them.

In May 1962 the South-west England faculty held a symposium in Torquay on General Practice premises. This was the first open discussion on the subject. In the meantime Dr Bruce Cardew had persuaded the General Medical Services Committee of the British Medical Association to sponsor an *ad hoc* group of representatives from that Committee, the College, the Medical Practitioners' Union, the Representative Body of the BMA and representatives of the Local Medical Committees. Its recommendation that the General Practice Advisory Service Limited should be established was accepted and work commenced in March 1964. This body could draw on the expertise accumulated by the College and took over the College's advisory service to general practitioners. Much work needed to be done as general practice was developing in many directions. The tendency for general practitioners to work in groups, using a single building, was being fostered and the first tentative steps were being taken to employ more receptionists, secretaries and nurses in these buildings.

In 1962 the committee came under the chairmanship of E. V. Kuenssberg and changed its role.

The continuation of operational research into many aspects of general practice resulted, among other things, in a publication on radio communication methods and their applicability to general practice. Work began on the standardization and prefabrication of general-practice premises and on their planning. Studies were carried out into the provision of General Medical Services in new towns and alternative forms of records for the National Health Service.

A further step was the setting up of courses in practice organization. Over the next few years this became a major part of the committee's work and courses were held throughout the British Isles.

THE NUFFIELD SURVEY

In 1961 the Nuffield Provincial Hospitals Trust sponsored an investigation into general practice. John Fry and J. B. Dillane with A. W. Lester, an architect, had been carrying out a pilot study into the conduct of general practice, its equipment and premises. With the aid of the Nuffield grant and the help of members of the committee this was expanded into a deeper study. Ann Cartwright and Rosalind Marshall of the Institute of Community Studies joined the committee. To begin with, ten practices were visited by John Dillane, Alfred Lester and George Adams to test its feasibility. Three separate studies followed:

(1) Fifty practices, randomly selected, were visited by the same team.

(2) Two hundred practices, again randomly selected, were circulated with a questionnaire designed to reveal how they conducted their practices and the equipment used.

(3) A percentage of the doctors who responded to the questionnaire were visited by Rosalind Marshall in order to expand some of the answers.

In 1964 the results of the survey were published under the title *General Practice Today, Its Conditions, Contents and Satisfaction,* by Ann Cartwright and Rosalind Marshall[3].

The Committee arranged an experimental weekend course on October 30–31 1965. This generated a demand from general practices all over the country. Three courses were held in London, two in Lancaster, and one each in Newcastle, Belfast, Leeds, Hull, Taunton and Glasgow and they were over subscribed.

The work expanded. Many faculties organized their own courses. Practice organization was an essential component of general-practitioner trainer courses. Course material and speakers were frequently supplied through the committee. Sixty to seventy per cent of the participants had introduced a new system of items of organization or equipment into their practices as a result of attending a course. So the committee had moved from being an operational research and advisory service unit to being the catalyst of education in practice organization.

In 1971, in its report to Council, the Committee noted:

The headquarters Practice Organization courses continue to be very popular. It was very encouraging to find on enquiry that practically every faculty has been running its own practice organization courses.

TEAM WORK

Over the years general practices had been increasing in size. From 1966 – the year of the Charter – onwards, most practices employed additional staff to help with both the clinical and administrative work. The Practice

Organization Committee responded to this challenge by evaluating modern organization and analysing the use of diagnostic equipment. This critical analysis included work done by nurses, health visitors, secretaries and receptionists. The study involved liaison with other organizations who nominated observers to the Committee. By 1972 the Central Council for the Education and Training of Health Visitors, the Society of Chief Nursing Officers, the British Association of Social Workers, the National Institute for Social-Work Training, the Department of Health and Social Security and the General Medical Services Committee of the BMA all sent observers and added greatly to the expertise of the Committee.

A document, *The Function of Ancillary Staff in General Practice,* appeared in 1970 and in revised form again in 1974. Other studies included *Function of the Physiotherapist in the Community, Computer Facilities and the Practitioner, The General Practitioner Team and the Community Hospital,* and *The Role of the Health Visitor.* Contacts were also developed with the Chartered Society of Physiotherapists and the Association of Medical Secretaries.

Conferences were held on some important subjects. The first of these was in 1966 organized in conjunction with the Office of Health Economics. It was devoted to the study of 'The Provision of General Medical Care in New Towns'[4]. The second conference took place on June 2 1966 and was on 'Studies of Buildings' by architects from the National Building Agency and the General Practice Advisory Service Limited; its report was published as the *Design Guide for Medical Group Practice Centres*[5], which became the local authorities' guide in this field. In 1969 a conference on 'Group Practice' was held under the chairmanship of J. E. Struthers. This gave rise to the publication *Group Practice Study Symposium.*

The early exhibitions of doctors' bags and instruments and the Exhibitions on Communications were all centred in London and, although this had many virtues, the College was always trying to 'get out to the periphery'. In 1966 a team of travelling lecturers from the Practice Organization Committee visited many parts of the United Kingdom and there was an exhibition of 'General Practice Tomorrow' which toured the seacoast of the UK in the yacht *Pharna,* sponsored by Nicholas Ltd and compiled by George Adams and Abraham Marcus.

Mary Hellier became Honorary Exhibition Secretary during 1967 and in 1968, with the co-operation and advice of various instrument firms and the generosity of Keeler Ltd and Allen and Hanbury Ltd, a permanent exhibition of instruments useful in general practice and domiciliary midwifery was set up and kept up-to-date. Suitable and appropriate exhibitions (e.g. electrocardiogram) which could be held at the College were arranged and were on view for about three months. An up-to-date display of catalogues, equipment and so on, was set up. Mobile exhibitions such as those on 'The Doctor's Bag' and 'Doctor's Premises' were designed and displayed with great help and encouragement, both financial and otherwise, from Mr Ellis Stanning of Lloyd Hamol Ltd.

PRACTICE ORGANIZATION STUDY

This Study was started in 1968 by Robin Ridsdill-Smith into the organization of general practice. It was well supported by members of the College who filled in the detailed questionnaire willingly, and supplied plans and photographs for inclusion in the books kept at 14 Princes Gate. This study proved to be a most useful source of knowledge and was improved in 1977 to identify innovations in general practice. A separate study was kept in the Exhibition Room.

The scope of exhibitions was steadily expanded. Apart from the Practice Organization Study, a series of major exhibitions was mounted, each lasting three to four months. The subjects were largely organizational and reflected the latest thinking in this field. They ranged from displays about practices to medical records and computers, from service medicine to health education. The display cabinets were changed every six months, in co-operation with Keeler Ltd, and displays concerning other College activities, for example, the Medical Recording Service and the Epidemic Observation Unit, were arranged. The Exhibition Service had a number of exhibits mounted on card for loan to faculties.

The year 1973 saw three publications which advanced general practice further. Austin Elliott and J. S. K. Stevenson produced one of the first blueprints from general practice for a health-care planning team on how to assess the geriatric needs of the community – *Geriatric Care in General Practice* [6]. The second edition of the *Design Guide* was produced – a reference work for architects and doctors engaged in the planning of new premises. A smaller study by Michael Drury on *Repeat Prescription Cards* [7] showed the increasing concern of the Committee with this topic.

1973 and 1974 were years of financial stringency. The Committee had grown greatly in size, because of increasing special interests of general practitioners. Two groups – one concerned mainly with forward studies and the other with liaison and co-operation – were formed. A further measure, resulting from the need to economize, was to see how much could be dealt with by post. The number of enquiries about aspects of practice organization coming in was growing each year.

The chairman of the Committee at that time, Michael Drury, invited Joan Mant and Barry Reedy to assess these enquiries and to make proposals. Their report was the seed from which the Central Information Service subsequently grew. During 1974 the number of enquiries reached 300 and, as many of these were on similar topics, a series of working papers was commissioned. During the next two or three years papers on A4 records the role of receptionists, practice nurses, practice managers and repeat prescriptions were prepared.

Under the auspices of the Kings' Fund, a working party was set up with A. Keable-Elliott as chairman; other members included James Cameron from the GMSC, Michael Drury and James Wood from the College, and representatives of Health Centre Administrators, the nursing services and the Department of Health and Social Security. This led to the establishment of the Central Information Service under the management of Joan Mant at the College, but supported by the GMSC and the DHSS.

References

1. Collings, J. S. (1950). General practice in England today. *Lancet,* **i**, 555–585
2. Taylor, S. (1954). *Good General Practice.* (London: Oxford University Press)
3. Cartwright, A. and Marshall, R. (1965). General practice in 1963: its conditions, contents and satisfaction. *Medical Care,* **3**, 69–87
4. Fry, J. and McKenzie, J. (eds.) (1967). *The Provision of General Medical Care in New Towns.* (London: Office of Health Economics)
5. College of General Practitioners and National Building Agency (1967). *Design Guide for Medical Group Practice Centres.* (London: NBA)
6. Elliott, A. E. and Stevenson, J. S. K. (1973). Geriatric care in general practice. *J. R. Coll. Gen. Practit.,* **23**, 615–625
7. Drury, V. W. M. (1973). Repeat prescription cards. *J. R. Coll. Gen. Practit.,* **23**, 511–514

XIII
COLLEGE PUBLICATIONS

THE ANNUAL REPORTS

John F. Burdon

Each year since the Foundation of the College an *Annual Report* of the College's work has been printed and sent to every fellow, member and associate with the agenda for the Annual General Meeting. These reports have proved to be a most valuable diary of College activities and an extremely helpful contribution to the dissemination of knowledge of the College's development during its first 25 years.

The number of printed pages in these relevant reports total approximately 3000 and describe the activities of the College, its Council and committees, its regional councils and faculties and their committees. Full details may be obtained by studying the reports themselves (copies of which are kept in the College library).

The editor of the *Annual Reports* up to 1958 was John Hunt, the honorary secretary of Council. He was joined by John F. Burdon, as assistant editor, in 1957, who took over the editorship in 1959. Annual reports of Council are constitutionally the responsibility of the honorary secretary of Council, and the College has been well served in this respect. Basil Slater took over from John Hunt in 1967 and was followed by Donald Irvine in 1972, whilst John Burdon continued as honorary editor.

In 1967 the *Annual Report* appeared with a new cover. A coat of arms had been printed in 1962 and now a space was made for the prefix 'Royal'. The portrait of John Hunt hanging in the Long Room at College headquarters shows him holding one of these reports – an indication of the value he and many others placed upon them as historical documents.

The 21st *Annual Report* (1973) found itself with the now familiar dark green and gilt jacket. This new look was generally approved as a suitable way to mark the College's coming of age.

In 1974 the financial report was included in the main body of the Report for the first time. The print order for the 25th *Annual Report* (1977) reached 9800. It had an appropriate silver cover to mark the anniversary.

THE COLLEGE JOURNAL

Denis J. Pereira Gray

The beginnings of the *Journal* (1953–54) are to be found in the activities of the Research Committee of the first Council of the College. Under the chairmanship of R. J. F. H. Pinsent, who was to remain on the *Journal*'s Editorial Board throughout the next 25 years, the Committee decided that to help fulfil Object E of the Memorandum of Association of the College,

> to encourage the publication by general medical practitioners of original work on medical and scientific subjects connected with general practice,

a newsletter should be produced which would appear quarterly and have a limited distribution. The first newsletter, consisting of cyclostyled sheets and marked 'Not for publication' appeared late in 1953.

EDITORSHIP OF R.M.S. MCCONAGHEY 1954–71

In 1954 it was decided that R. M. S. McConaghey, a member of the Foundation Council and of the first Research Committee, should become editor of the *Newsletter* which he then proceeded to develop from his home in Dartmouth, Devon. His Editorial Board consisted of G. F. Abercrombie, D. G. French, J. H. Hunt, R. J. F. H. Pinsent and G. I. Watson, all of whom were members of the Foundation Council. His first issue appeared in October 1954. At the beginning of 1955 he introduced a new format with *Research Newsletter No 6*. During 1955 and 1956 the material in the *Newsletter* gradually changed from being devoted entirely to research to reporting much of the work of the growing College and increasingly about general practice itself.

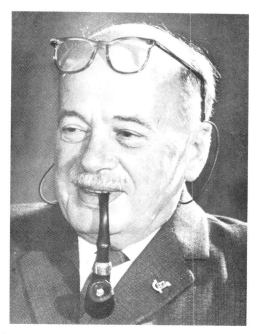

Plate 11 R. M. S. McConaghey, Founder Editor of the *Journal* of the College and Editor from 1958 to 1971

Newsletter to Journal

In January 1958, for the first time R. M. S. McConaghey introduced the word *Journal* into the title which thus became *Journal of the College of General Practitioners*. At the same time he removed the words 'Not for publication' from the cover. In the editorial of the same issue, tribute was paid to *The Practitioner* and to the *Medical World* which 'have gone out of their way to encourage the general practitioner to publish his views'. It is interesting to see how defensive the *Journal* was at that time: 'Whilst it may be argued that there are already too many journals being contributed to by too many authors, the general practitioner has in the past often found it difficult to get his views published'[1].

The pattern was established. A quarterly journal, guided by the same Editorial Board and offering an increasing number and range of interests began. Reports of annual meetings appeared, also lists of members of Council, new members of the College, and numerous clinical reports.

In 1960 the pages were sewn for the first time instead of stapled, thus producing a flat spine. The old *Research Newsletter* title was dropped altogether and John F. Burdon of Paignton became Assistant Editor.

When the College received its coat of arms in 1962, the *Journal* reproduced it on the cover with the motto '*Cum Scientia Caritas*'. The same year M. I. Cookson and G. Swift joined the Board and the subscription, which had previously been one guinea a year for four issues or six shillings a copy, was raised to two guineas or seven and sixpence a copy.

An important change took place in 1964 when the *Journal* started to appear in alternate months, producing six issues a year instead of four.

Two years later M. J. Linnett and I. R. McWhinney joined the Board and when the College became 'Royal' in 1967, the new title appeared for the first time on the cover of the May issue. New members of the Editorial Board that year were W. G. Keane and J. F. Burdon.

Monthly Journal

The big step to monthly publication was taken in 1968. The subscription went up to four guineas a year. For the first time the *Journal* was now published by professional publishers, E. & S. Livingstone of Edinburgh, although it retained the same printers, the Devonshire Press Ltd of Torbay.

The Editorial Board was increased in size to include D. J. Pereira Gray, R. M. Griffiths, B. C. S. Slater, I. H. Stokoe and J. R. Miles.

In January 1969 the *Journal*'s white cover gave way to blue and the number of pages increased to 60. This format was retained until the end of R. M. S. McConaghey's editorship on December 31 1971.

Assessment

The early history of the *Journal* has already been analysed by Murray Scott (1970)[1], and assessments have been made of McConaghey's editorship[2,3].

Dr McConaghey's achievement was unique. He created from a private cyclostyled newsletter a scientific medical journal for his discipline. He had the foresight to concentrate on original rather than review articles. For a period of 17 years he edited the *Journal* while continuing in general practice in Dartmouth, resolutely pursuing his ideals in both jobs. His period of office, during which he edited 117 issues of the *Journal* and 30 associated publications, may never be surpassed.

In 1975, a month before his death but with his knowledge and appreciation, his name was added to the title page of the *Journal* in perpetuity, as Founding Editor. It has been said of him as a man that:

He stood on the classic tripod of the family doctor – being happy at home, proud of his practice, and contented in his community. . . . Ahead of his time, he foresaw before it happened that general practitioners would increasingly report original research from general practice itself. He deliberately fashioned an instrument of communication which would foster the highest standards and would appropriately represent his discipline. He was greatly helped and loyally supported by the *Journal*'s first business manager, Miss Irene Scawn. He strove for quality rather than quantity, and the *Journal* became the academic voice of general practice. . . . As an honorary part-time medical editor he broke new ground. His achievement was unique and made him the leading part-time medical editor in the Western world. McConaghey was for the part-timers what Fox and Garland represent for the professionals[3].

EDITORSHIP OF D. J. PEREIRA GRAY 1972–1980

D. J. Pereira Gray, a member of the Editorial Board since 1968, was appointed Deputy Editor in December 1970, and succeeded to the Editorship on January 1 1972. The *Journal* office moved to Exeter and the *Journal* was edited from his home, supported by a full-time secretary and his wife as half-time editorial assistant. She had had previous experience in journalism.

A new Editorial Board was appointed to include a number of younger doctors. Its composition was: John Hunt, D. H. Irvine, E. V. Kuenssberg, M. L. Marinker, G. N. Marsh, J. R. Miles, R. J. F. H. Pinsent, G. I. Watson and H. J. Wright.

Change of Publishers

In the summer of 1976 Council of the College decided to change publishers and move to Update Publications Ltd. This led to a change of printers and the *Journal* was now printed by Cradleys of Cradley Heath, Warwickshire. The format changed to international size A4, and a substantial increase in the number of advertisements was obtained.

During the 1970s new members of the Editorial Board were S. L. Barley, H. W. K. Acheson, S. J. Carne, D. G. Garvie, J. C. Hasler, C. Waine and Professor J. S. McCormick. In 1978 J. R. Miles, R. J. F. H. Pinsent and G. I. Watson retired, the last two after unbroken membership of the Editorial Board since the *Journal*'s foundation.

Philosophy

R. M. S. McConaghey's achievement had been to establish a journal of general practice where there had been none before. Denis Pereira Gray, who always acknowledged and greatly appreciated the help he had received from his predecessor, saw as his role its development and expansion.

He saw the College *Journal* developing to become the *British Journal of General Practice* and this title was adopted as the subtitle in January 1976.

One of the problems of the early years had been that in its attempt to establish standards the *Journal* had become somewhat remote and was not being widely read and discussed. He believed that such a journal must be read, even if people disagreed with its contents, and he was particularly concerned that it should seem interesting and challenging to young principals and trainees.

The changes introduced hinged on his confidence in the future both of general practice as a whole, and of the College and the *Journal* in particular. He felt both were now strong enough to withstand challenge and criticism which he began to encourage. Criticisms of general practice were now met head on and the decision to publish Honigsbaum's (1972) critique[4], although bitterly resented by some at the time, reflected the determination of many in general practice to face their critics openly with the aim of raising standards.

Articles

A scientific journal must primarily be judged by the quality of the articles which it publishes. During the 1970s there was a steady change as the number and quality of articles in the *Journal* rose, almost imperceptibly at first but later more rapidly. At the beginning of the 1970s the *Journal* often received articles rejected by other journals, but by the end of the decade papers were appearing in journals all over the world which had previously been rejected by the College *Journal*. Articles began to be published which were widely quoted within general practice and later outside it as well.

About a dozen editorials in the *British Medical Journal* and *The Lancet* were devoted to papers which had appeared in the College *Journal* or its associated publications, and the *Journal*'s articles became internationally accepted as standard references.

Certain general themes emerged during the decade. First, the medico-sociological influence became apparent with major contributions from authors like Margot Jeffreys, Ann Cartwright and psychiatrists and psychologists from the Tavistock Institute. Another important trend was education, especially postgraduate training in which the Editor was particularly concerned as a part-time senior lecturer in general practice at Exeter. A third trend was medical audit and quality of care, with slow but gradually increasing emphasis on ordinary clinical work in general practice.

At the beginning of the 1970s most articles about general practice gave references to other medical journals; by the end of the 1970s it was rare to have an important article on general practice that did not carry a reference to the College *Journal*. In some subjects, especially audit, medical education and the behavioural aspects of medicine, the *Journal* had emerged as the main academic source.

An early decision of the Editorial Board in 1972 was to encourage authorship by young principals and vocational trainees. In the early 1970s many articles had to be rejected, but with extensive assistance of the Editorial Board more and more were found suitable for publication. By 1977 the *Journal* was publishing every two or three months one article by a trainee practitioner[5].

During the decade an ever increasing amount of time and effort was devoted to reshaping and improving the presentation of articles in the *Journal*. Many went to and fro between the author and the *Journal* office three or four times before final acceptance. More and more time was spent on shortening and editing the text and reorganizing tables and figures. Summaries were introduced, and a formal system of headings to conform to accepted standards for original research.

Whereas Dr McConaghey had struggled for years to insist on an appropriate use of references – a battle which was well won by the time of his retirement – Denis Pereira Gray's struggle was with statistics. He insisted on a more professional approach from authors and made increasing use of professional statisticians and epidemiologists as advisers in order to raise standards.

The number of the editorials increased, with an average of about two an issue. The range broadened to include clinical, organizational, educational, social and general topical comment on developments in medicine and general practice. Some modern journalistic techniques were introduced, particularly alliterative headings and a questioning rather than a didactic style. The *Journal* no longer avoided controversy and where there was more than one side, stated both but did not hide its own preference. The tribute to Michael Balint[6] in March 1972, for example, concluded: 'What Freud has become for psychiatry, Balint will become for general practice'.

The editorials began to attract comments not just from medical journals but from the national press. *The Times,* the *Daily Telegraph*, the *Guardian*, as well as all the medical journals, increasingly published articles or quotations based on *Journal* editorials.

Letters to the Editor

Murray Scott (1970)[1] wrote that the correspondence column had 'never proved very lively' but the editorial policy of accepting criticism and challenging the *status quo* meant that the opposite soon became true. The Editor saw himself as neutral in the inevitable tension between the College establishment and its critics and considered that the *Journal* should be an open forum in which the most junior associate could and should be able to criticize College policy and the senior Officers of the College should always have a right of reply.

Despite the inherent difficulties of monthly publication, the number of letters increased to such an extent that many had to be shortened and numbers restricted. Under a new heading of 'Letters to the Editor' a sharp, entertaining, and lively column ensued.

Other Features

The quantity and proportion of factual information was increased by an expansion of the news section which, in addition to College news, sought to provide general information about events in British medicine and in general practice in particular. Signed book reviews were introduced in 1973 and have been continued ever since.

Private Subscriptions

Denis Pereira Gray always believed that the *Journal* should be supported by a large income from private subscriptions, which would underpin academic independence. He inherited 379 private subscriptions at £5.25 each and an annual subscription income of under £2000 a year. These steadily increased over the years.

Journal Publications

Journal publications consist of a series of separate booklets all of which were not only edited but also published by the College *Journal* office. Denis Pereira Gray edited and published three *Reports from General Practice (Nos 15–17)* and 10 *Supplements*. In 1976 he started the new *Occasional Paper* series.

By late 1977 over 1000 copies of *Occasional Papers* were sold from 14 Princes Gate, and the series appears established for the future. The topics have varied widely from practice organization and research classification, to sociological studies and medical education.

Continuing Evolution of the Journal

The College *Journal* by its nature and style will always reflect not only the development of the College itself, but of the whole discipline of general practice. Although the balance of content will vary, it will always reflect current interests of the profession, and the Editor and the Editorial Board will focus the topics like a magnifying glass. Not only does such a *Journal* chart the evolution of the main changes in general practice, it also reveals the pace of those changes. Broad trends in the development of general practice can be seen by analysis of its pages. It is clear, for example, that in the 1950s the College and its foundation members were preoccupied with its early development.

In the 1960s this was followed by a wave of interest and writing about practice organization, which was succeeded in its turn by education, especially specific postgraduate vocational training for general practice.

The *Journal* is the principal means of communication between the College and its members. It has been throughout the life of the College, like the *Annual Report,* a service which has reached every fellow, member and associate of the College without exception wherever he lives. For many it is the one and only contact with the College and with other College members, and it has therefore a special significance. Its value in the dissemination of news and ideas is paramount and it has done much throughout the last quarter century to keep the College members in touch with each other and to preserve and develop the consensus of policy-making which has been a feature of the College during this time.

Quite apart, however, from the significance of the *Journal* to College members, it has an especially important and often underrated significance to those outside the College, outside general practice, and outside the United Kingdom. It is widely read abroad and talked about and quoted in countries throughout the English-speaking world.

To doctors outside general practice, both in departments of government and in other branches of medicine, the *Journal* has become the voice of general practice. It is the visible evidence of the determination of general practice to put its own house in order, to improve standards, and above all to encourage original research in its own discipline and for medicine as a whole.

167

OTHER COLLEGE PUBLICATIONS

Denis J. Pereira Gray

Throughout its first 25 years, the Royal College of General Practitioners has always been a minority body, although latterly a large one; even in 1977 only about a third of British general practitioners were members. In tracing the history of the College's influence, the *Journal* and College publications must rank high as among the means whereby the College has communicated its ideas to the medical world.

REPORTS FROM GENERAL PRACTICE

The *Reports from General Practice* are a series of separate publications published by the *Journal* which either represent College policy or at least carry College approval. The first of these, *Special Vocational Training,* was issued with the Journal in May 1965, price five shillings. It was quite small, consisting of only 26 pages, and carried the words 'Published by the Council of the College of General Practitioners'. Although the idea of special training for general practice was first suggested by the Cohen Committee in 1950, it was this little booklet that reported the decision of W. H. Hylton's committee, whose membership included two future presidents of the College, a chairman of Council and two regional advisers, which had a truly dramatic effect. Although little else happened between 1950 and 1965 on this subject, within 11 years of the publication of the report, the National Health Service (Vocational Training) Act 1976 was passed by Parliament, which gave authority for four years' compulsory training for general practice after qualification.

There is no space to comment individually on the other *Reports from General Practice,* except to note that education and training have been the dominant themes. *Number 5* was the published Evidence of the Royal College to the Royal Commission on Medical Education, which was almost completely accepted and opened the doors for the dramatic advances in vocational training in the following years. Undoubtedly it was the influence on the Royal Commission on Medical Education in its 1968 report (the Todd Report) and the College's well-publicized arguments for special training for general practice which led to the Conference of Local Medical Committees adopting the policy which hoped to persuade government to introduce legislation.

Number 6, The Implementation of Vocational Training; Number 11, The General Practitioner Teaching of Undergraduates in British Medical Schools; Number 15, Teaching Practices; and *Number 17, The Assessment of Vocational Training for General Practice,* all followed the training theme and were written either by a College committee or by leading College educationalists.

One other important series stands out: *The Present State and Future Needs of General Practice* series, which was planned and coordinated by John Fry, first published in 1965 and reaching a third edition in 1973. The extent of this work subsequently became so great that a book, *Trends in General Practice,* took the place of a fourth edition (see below).

In summary, the influence of the *Reports from General Practice* series has been truly remarkable and has extended far beyond the small emerging College which produced them.

BOOKS AND OTHER PUBLICATIONS

Three other early publications by the College each had considerable influence. *Studies on Medical and Population Subjects, No 14,* was the first of the *Morbidity Statistics from General Practice* series: volume three was written by the College (HMSO, 1958–62). The College collaborated with the National Building Agency in producing the *Design Guide for Medical Group Practice Centres* in 1967 which has influenced many practice buildings all over the country. Thirdly, the publication *Family Health Care – The Team* (1967) reported on collaboration between general practitioners and colleagues in the other caring professions.

The Future General Practitioner – Learning and Teaching

At the beginning of the 1970s the College formed an outstanding team led by John Horder as chairman and consisting of Patrick Byrne, Donald Irvine, Conrad Harris, Paul Freeling and Marshall Marinker, to produce what was then known as the *Fourth Report.* Published by the *British Medical Journal* on behalf of the College in 1972, this must rank as the most important and so far the most successful of all the College's books. It included on page 1 an important job definition and provided the first formal presentation in English of the content of general practice with some guidelines as to how it could be taught. Of particular importance for the future was the acceptance of educational theory and the couching of the book in educational terms including aims and objectives. This has provided the first published framework for the vocational training courses which subsequently sprang up all over the British Isles. The book has stood the test of time. It has already been translated into several languages and been reprinted on numerous occasions. The profits go to the College Appeal.

Epidemiology in Country Practice

W. N. Pickles has been widely revered by British general practitioners and his *Epidemiology in Country Practice,* first published in 1939, was a masterpiece recognized throughout the world. Unfortunately it went out of print, but thanks to the inspiration of R. M. S. McConaghey, the copyright was secured and a special facsimile leatherbound edition was printed by the Devonshire Press Ltd of Torbay. A limited edition of 1000 copies was produced (1970) and sold, the profits going to the College Appeal. Although this book did not have College authorship, Pickles was the first President of the College and the venture serves to illustrate another role played by the College in disseminating and making more widely available a text which would not otherwise have been printed at the time.

Morbidity Statistics from General Practice

The Report of the *Second Study on Morbidity Statistics from General Practice 1970–71* was published in 1974 as No 26 in the *Studies on Medical Population Series* by HM Stationery Office. The three organizations responsible for the work were the Royal College of General Practitioners, the Office of Population Censuses and Surveys and the Department of Health and Social Security. The ideas had been developed by the College, notably the diagnostic register ('E' Book). The records for the practices were cross-checked in detail by staff from the Office of Population Censuses and Surveys and the study was carried out as thoroughly as any morbidity recording in Europe at that time. The work stands as an important yardstick of morbidity in general practice, and as a national and international reference. It is to be hoped that the system will be continued in the next decade so that future changes in morbidity can be identified.

Oral Contraceptives and Health

In the same year, *Oral Contraceptives and Health* was published as an interim report from the Oral Contraception Study of the Manchester Research Unit of the Royal College of General Practitioners, directed by Clifford Kay. It was published by Pitman Medical and recorded the largest single prospective trial of a prescribed product carried out anywhere in the world. In the foreword, HRH The Prince Philip, Duke of Edinburgh, Patron and Immediate Past President of the College, wrote that

Since 1968, 1400 general practitioners and about 46 000 women had been involved in this long-term study in which the results were computerized. Although further research will be needed and the oral contraception study itself is continuing, there can be no doubt that this work stands as a milestone in the development of multi-disciplinary practice recording and it pioneered important principles of confidentiality. In multi-practice research, the system of using controls selected from age/sex registers in the same practice and under the care of the same doctors in the same area has proved valuable and is an important method for the future.

Trends in General Practice 1977

A recent book published by the College, *Trends in General Practice 1977*, grew out of the *Present State and Future Needs* series which had first appeared as *Reports from General Practice* with the *Journal*. It consisted of a series of essays by selected members of the College, under the general editorship of John Fry, and was produced by the *British Medical Journal* in the same format as *The Future General Practitioner*. The book has been widely read and has become a popular reference. It is used particularly by doctors preparing for the membership examination of the College.

FACULTY PUBLICATIONS

John F. Burdon

The records from which this account was compiled were obtained partly from replies to a circular letter sent out to honorary secretaries of faculty boards and partly from index cards held by the librarian at Princes Gate. A mass of data, minutes, papers, journals and letters was assembled, and it became quite evident that the compilation of a history of faculty publications was not simple. And this was from replies from only 11 of the 35 faculties circulated!

It is not possible to state that faculties which did not reply did not have newsletters or other publications, but positive evidence of newsletter production came from 18 faculties. These publications varied in style and content, being sometimes mere circulars, and sometimes in letterpress thanks to the assistance of certain pharmaceutical houses. Advertisements were noteworthy by their absence.

Some faculties sent their newsletters to all trainees in their area (e.g. East Anglia), and some circulated to all NHS general practitioners via the Family Practitioner Committee's mailing, thus economizing on postage to pay for the extra copies needed (e.g. Essex and South-east Scotland).

The 800 or so reports from faculties already published in the *Annual Reports* of the College for the first 25 years mention many other publications or subjects which have been discussed by faculties.

References

1. Scott, R. A. M. (1970). The development of the College Journal. *J. R. Coll. Gen. Practit.,* **20,** 255–262
2. *Journal of the Royal College of General Practitioners* (1972). R. M. S. McConaghey. **22,** 1–4
3. *Journal of the Royal College of General Practitioners* (1975). Mac. **25,** 627–629
4. Honigsbaum, F. (1972). Quality in general practice. *J. R. C. Gen. Practit.,* **22,** 429–451
5. *Journal of the Royal College of General Practitioners* (1979). Trainee projects. **29,** 452–455
6. *Journal of the Royal College of General Practitioners* (1972). **22,** 133–135

XIV
THE LIBRARY, MUSEUM AND ARCHIVES

PART I: THE LIBRARY

Michael J. Linnett and Margaret Hammond

After the death of Dr Geoffrey Evans, his library, with a handsome bookcase, was presented to the College and formed the nucleus of the College Library. A room in the new headquarters was set aside for the collection, and Council agreed that it should be named *The Geoffrey Evans Library*. John Horder, who had previously been appointed College Archivist by Council, was appointed the first Honorary Librarian to the College, and Michael Linnett Honorary Assistant Librarian.

After widespread consultations a summary of opinions on the object and contents of the College Library was prepared by John Horder for presentation to the first meeting of the Library Committee of Council on October 29 1958, at which Lindsey Batten was elected chairman. The Committee's terms of reference were

To advise and assist Council on all matters relating to books, archives and other objects of historical interest.

At this meeting objectives were established. They were that the Library should eventually contain, firstly, everything written about general practice and, secondly, everything written on medical subjects by general practitioners. Reprints of members' works were to be collected, the librarian had discretion to purchase other books subject to the approval of the Library Committee and, later, a small number of standard reference books in other branches of medicine was added.

It was decided, also, that the Library should represent the interests of the College to visitors and that recent publications, especially the published works of the College and its members, should be displayed in it. It should be used for reference by visiting members and staff; but it should not lend books outside the building. These principles and objectives have governed the work of the Library up to the present day.

Standing Committees of Council were asked to suggest books and periodicals which the Library should contain. Within the first year a large number of gifts had been received, the beginning of a flow of books of medical and historical interest, collections of periodicals and so on.

The librarians of other institutions – the British Medical Association, the Royal College of Physicians, the Royal College of Surgeons, the Royal Society of Medicine and the Wellcome Historical Medical Library – were generous with their encouragement, help and advice. In particular Mr John L. Thornton, librarian of St Bartholomew's Hospital Medical College, was unstinting in guiding and helping, in a most practical way, the developing Library; he was invited to become Consultant Librarian to the College. He filled this office with distinction until he retired. With his advice a start was made on a catalogue of the collection of books, journals and other documents, particularly those concerned with the founding of the College.

Photocopying Service

A notable addition to the library service occurred in 1959, when John Wyeth and Brother Ltd generously offered the sum of £750 yearly to fund the purchase and operation of a photocopying machine. With the generous co-operation of the Librarian of the Royal College of Surgeons, Mr W. R. le Fanu, the machine was installed for over ten years at the Library of that College, whose enormous collection of some 500 current journals served as the main source of the documents requested by our members and associates. Through this scheme members have been able to obtain from the Library, at little or no expense, copies of any articles in which they were specially interested. This flow of information stimulated interest in other aspects of the Library's work. The Wyeth grant also meant that a part-time librarian could be appointed.

College Librarians

On June 1 1960 the College's first professional librarian, Mrs Rosemary Rabé, ALA, started work. With her arrival there was a great expansion of the service available through the library to members, notably in searches

174

through the literature to produce the subject bibliographies that have become such a feature of the Library. Because of this growth in activities it soon became necessary to employ a part-time worker to deal solely with the photocopying requirements; and during the next three years it became clear that a full-time librarian was essential.

In 1963 Miss Margaret Hammond, who trained in medical librarianship at St Bartholomew's Hospital and at Guy's Hospital, was appointed Librarian. This proved a wise choice, for under her direction the College Library has prospered and expanded to achieve the international reputation it enjoys today.

Bibliographies, Lists and Catalogues

A grant from the Royal Society in 1964 was followed by another from the Usher Institute in Edinburgh which helped to establish a list of as many research projects concerning general practice as could be found. By 1967 the first edition of *Research Projects by General Practitioners* was published and was followed by several other editions.

Meanwhile an extensive catalogue of library contents, books, journals and papers, was built up to provide a readily available source of reference for members, and even for outside bodies. Concurrently the collection of subject bibliographies was extended and kept up-to-date so that it became possible to supply any member with references relevant to a given subject within a few days. Since 1964 some 5500 bibliographies have been prepared – around 400 each year.

Gifts

In 1970 the College acquired a notable collection of papers and documents left by William Pickles, the first President of the College. This gift is described in more detail in Part III of this chapter (Archives). Together these items form a unique record of the work of this remarkable general practitioner. Many other collections of papers have been acquired, including a gift from Sir John Parkinson of letters written by Sir James Mackenzie.

Honorary Librarian

In 1971 Denis Craddock was appointed Honorary Librarian. He had played an important part in selecting books for the Library when it was started, and had himself written extensively. Under his guidance the Library was able to respond to the different demands made of it by the proliferating work and influence of the College, both nationally and internationally.

'New Reading'

The development of vocational training schemes and postgraduate centres, particularly in the 1970s, produced a special emphasis on education. Trainees needed up-to-date information on new publications about general practice and work related to it. To meet this need in 1975 the Library started to produce a quarterly publication, *New Reading for General Practitioners*, a list of books and papers arranged under subject headings from the material seen in the Library. With the advent of systematic training for general practice this publication has become an important teaching tool for Regional Advisers and Course Organizers.

British Library Computer Terminal Reference Service (BLAISE)

The new generation of technology, with the availability of the British Library Computer Terminal Reference Service (BLAISE), and the use of microfiche in the storage of an increasing number of journals, will inevitably mean changes in library techniques with, it is hoped, an expansion of the services that the Library can provide for the College.

PART II: THE MUSEUM

Peter Thomas

Winston Churchill realized how essential the past was in relation to the present and future when, in an address to the Royal College of Physicians in 1944, he said 'The longer you can look back, the further you can look forward'. He was so right. Douglas Guthrie, the eminent Scottish laryngologist and medical historian, always stressed the need for a knowledge of the origin of one's profession. He reminded us very forcibly that medical history is not, in any sense, a special branch of medicine. One way in which our College could acquire this knowledge (apart from the spoken or written word) lay in the founding of a museum where emphasis could be laid on the visual approach to further our studies.

The history of our Museum is co-extensive with the history of the

College itself. A discerning Foundation Council was quick to stress the importance of collecting, preserving and displaying rare items, both old and contemporary, relating specifically to general practice in its widest sense and also to medical history in general. The business of the Museum was delegated to the Library Committee of Council. Constant appeals to College members and associates over the years for objects of historic interest have led to a generous response not only from our own membership but also from the public. A response truly reflecting man's love of the past and his innate desire to conserve the vital evidence necessary for a valid interpretation of his own professional and cultural evolution.

In 1959, Peter Thomas was appointed Honorary Curator and, with the generous support of successive librarians and staff, he continues to serve in that capacity.

In the early years he sought and received much help from university departments and other educational centres in order to gain information about the promotion of the idea. Noteworthy in this respect was the contribution of the Wellcome Historical Medical Museum. From that Foundation, Dr Margaret Rowbottom and Mr J. W. Barber-Lomax not only proffered valuable practical advice from time to time but were instrumental in donating five showcases for the use of the College at Princes Gate. The purchase of showcases has always been a problem to any developing institution as their cost has been prohibitive. To be given five such cabinets at once was a tremendous boost to our ability to arrange displays in rotation under secure conditions.

During the past 20 years the work of cataloguing the wide variety of museum objects has continued steadily. When the College was 25 years old the collection consisted of upwards of 500 items or groups of items, one of the earliest being a Culpeper-type microscope dating from the late eighteenth century. The bulk of the material, including surgical and medical instruments, old textbooks, documents, prescription books, qualifying certificates and diplomas, drug jars, prints etc, belongs to the nineteenth century. The early twentieth century is represented by several Dudgeon's sphygmographs and Mackenzie polygraphs used by general practitioners half a century ago. The range of accessions can only be appreciated by recourse to the museum index kept up-to-date by Miss Margaret Hammond and Mrs Lorna Neale. It is also noteworthy that the second College Archivist, Alastair Murray Scott, gave generously of his time in restoring some of the wooden instrument cases to their former glory.

The museum has a loan function also. The Curator and Librarian are willing to consider requests for historical material for display on stands and at exhibitions, provided security arrangements are satisfactory. It has been suggested that every faculty should appoint its own honorary curator, whose duties might include those of archivist also. He could direct and coordinate all action in relation to antiquarian matters in the faculty area in a unique way.

Musarum templa colamus.

PART III: THE ARCHIVES*

John Horder and Alastair Murray Scott

The appointment of an Archivist was first raised in Council in December 1955 by Annis Gillie and Robin Pinsent. A decision was postponed until 1956, when the matter was brought up again by John Henderson. John Horder, who had prepared a discussion paper, was appointed as the College's first Archivist. Alastair Murray Scott succeeded as Archivist in 1968.

The rightness of the decision to collect archives was confirmed by a comment of Mr L.E. Payne, the Librarian of the Royal College of Physicians; he deeply regretted that his College had not formally established a collection of archives until long after its foundation.

Chairmen and honorary secretaries of central and faculty committees were asked to submit material which they were ready to discard. Many did this. The Research Committee was notably assiduous. It was in 1968 that it was decided to examine their collection of letters, agendas and reports. They were determined not to lose anything of value to the future historian, and had stored all such communications since the start of research work, that is, for about 15 years. These papers were packed into a number of large cartons and sent to headquarters. The task of sorting fell to the new Archivist and entailed many pleasant, though occasionally boring, visits to headquarters. At those times when the work seemed merely to be the filling of wastepaper baskets the cheerful and helpful presence of Margaret Hammond, the Librarian, always made the visit worthwhile. During 18 months much material of historical, social and scientific interest was filed in the archives.

In 1969 William Pickles, the first President, died and, with the willing help of his daughter, Patricia Clayton, and her husband, much material of great personal and general interest was collected. Items such as a specimen diary taken on his rounds, charts and clinical records, typescripts of more

---

* 'Documents produced and preserved in the course of business, as distinct from publications (library or material collected for its own sake).'

than 20 lectures, a large collection of reprints, stethoscope and thermometer and certificates of honorary degrees and medals went to the College archives, museum and library.

In 1977 Geoffrey Sykes of the Yorkshire faculty suggested to Council that, as well as letters, minutes and reports, it might consider compiling a list of members who would be qualified to talk on the foundation of the College and who could produce a live record for the archives on tape. The archivist thereupon contacted all living foundation members, asking each for a curriculum vitae or potted biography, stressing in particular his or her reason for joining the College, and arranging for a tape record of the voices of those not already in the archives. The four unrecorded members assembled at Headquarters and, with the help of the Graves Audiovisual Service and the able prompting of John Lawson, produced a memorable tape for the archives.

To these voices can be added those of the many lecturers and speakers at College symposia. To give life to these voices the archives had a considerable number of photographs of College members taken by enthusiasts, many of which are up to professional standard, especially those of Ivor Cookson. Several of these are in this book.

Alongside this main collection, inevitably patchy in scope, there are two other important sources of archive material – the bound volumes of minutes of Council and Committees kept since 1953; and papers in the possession of Lord Hunt of Fawley which may prove to be the most important source for the earliest part of the College's history.

The original decision to establish Archives subsequently led to the start of a Library at the College in 1957.

XV
HEADQUARTERS, STAFF AND ADMINISTRATION

John H. Hunt (1952–77) *and James Wood* (1971–77)

MANSFIELD STREET (1952)

The first headquarters of the College were at 7 Mansfield Street, London W1. This was a house owned by Dr Geoffrey Evans, a general consulting physician and senior physician of St Bartholomew's Hospital. He had always shown a particular interest in the problems of general practice. He taught me a great deal of medicine, I contributed to his book on Medical Treatment, and we became good friends.

In the autumn of 1951, just before anyone began to think seriously about how to form a new College, Dr Evans died suddenly and tragically as the result of an accident at his country home. His family asked me to write his obituary notice in *The Times*. When our Steering Committee was being formed, Mrs Evans and her son, Ancrum, offered us for our meetings the use of a large room on the ground floor of their house. It was the patients' waiting room and the family's dining room where, for many years, family prayers had been held each morning. Most of the meetings of the Steering Committee took place in that pleasant room, including the historic eighth and last when the College was founded and the first meeting of the Provisional Foundation Council which followed immediately. This house was central, convenient and fairly easily reached by Henry Willink who came by car from Cambridge.

For a few weeks in 1953, just after the College had been founded and the Steering Committee's report had been published, we were invited to use the room at 7 Mansfield Street as an office. During those few weeks more than 1000 doctors from many parts of the world joined our young College.

181

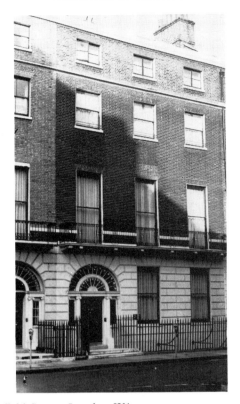

Plate 12   7 Mansfield Street, London W1

Sylvia Chapman came to us as Honorary Registrar, a post she held for many years. She was very busy during those first few weeks at Mansfield Street acknowledging application forms, receipting entrance fees, and ensuring that applicants conformed to the simple criteria for entrance to membership which had been laid down at that time. Very soon she had an assistant.

Shortly afterwards the Evans family sold 7 Mansfield Street and College Headquarters moved to 54 Sloane Street, London SW1, the house from which I practised.

SLOANE STREET (1953–1957)

Here the College occupied a large bright room on the first floor facing west with a small side room. Members of the College were welcome during office

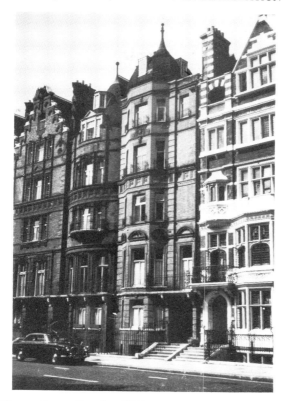

Plate 13   54 Sloane Street, London SW1

hours to talk to Dr Chapman and inspect the maps and registers concerned with the early development of the College and its regional faculties. The nucleus of our College Library was there too – the first of the books presented to us by the executors of the late Dr Geoffrey Evans. Office furniture, files, typewriters, a dictaphone transcriber and a duplicating machine had to be bought. A full-time and a part-time secretary were employed to help with all Dr Chapman's work.

One secretary had been warmly recommended to us as a most efficient, honest and reliable person by a consultant member of the Steering Committee. Unfortunately this turned out not to be the case; she was taken to court and convicted of forging our signatures on a great many cheques and stealing a considerable sum of the College's money. She went to prison for this and other offences. The Bank repaid us in full and with interest. The forged signatures were poor facsimiles of the originals.

After this sad and upsetting affair we employed a senior administrative secretary – Commander A. E. P. Doran DSC, RN (Retd.) whom George Abercrombie found for us through his naval connections. Peter Doran served us well for many years. Mrs Eileen Phillips had been my secretary in practice a year or so before, until she had been taken ill. When recovered, she also joined us in the College office, and a very efficient, hard-working and faithful employee she proved to be during the next 16 years. She was friendly, charming, one of the fastest and most accurate typists I have met; she had the welfare of the College deeply at heart and nothing was too much trouble for her. The College owed her a great debt. We made her an Honorary Fellow in May 1971.

Number 54 Sloane Street had a large hall with a high ceiling. In the autumn of 1957 a few weeks before the College's Annual General Meeting this hall was packed full to the ceiling with post-office sacks containing large envelopes addressed to about 4000 members and associates, containing agenda, other notices and the *Annual Report*. One afternoon on seeing this a patient said to me: 'I notice that you are sending out your bills!'

After five years the two rooms at Sloane Street became much too small for the work which had, by then, to be done. So we moved on March 17 1958 to 41 Cadogan Gardens, London SW3, opposite the west side of Peter Jones.

CADOGAN GARDENS (1958–1962)

This move was made possible through the kindness of Mr Reginald Graham, a patient of mine, who leased it and let us use it at a nominal rent. He repaired and redecorated the premises and gave us some furniture, including a fine desk. We were very grateful to him. This house was large enough to hold all the equipment and secretarial staff which we had then.

A room at the back was just large enough to hold a council meeting, although nearly all meetings of Council and its Committees still took place in the beautiful Court Room and Hall of the Worshipful Society of Apothecaries, Black Friars Lane, by kind permission of its Master and Court. In 1969 the College presented that Society with a fine silver Armada Dish (see Chapter III).

41 Cadogan Gardens, London SW3, was the first registered office of our 'Incorporated College', under the Companies' Act 1948. The certificate dated February 8 1961 was laid on the table at the first Council Meeting of the Incorporated College held on March 26 1961.

We were at 41 Cadogan Gardens for five years, an important period of consolidation during which all the College activities still steadily increased.

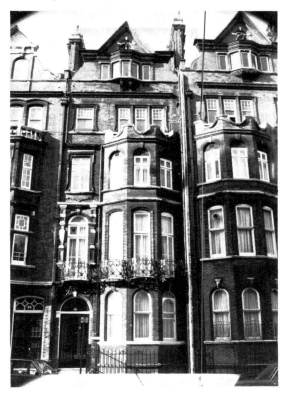

Plate 14   41 Cadogan Gardens, London SW3

At the end of that time this house also became too small and, although Mr Graham had generously extended the lease, Council decided that we should try to find a large building near the centre of London, if possible freehold, which we could buy as a permanent home for our rapidly developing young College.

PRINCES GATE (1963–1977)

For many months the search went on. Several possible sites were carefully considered. One was at the corner of Cavendish Square and Queen Anne Street, another a large leasehold block next door to the Royal College of Surgeons in Lincoln's Inn Fields and a third was the Incorporated Accountant's Hall on the Embankment near the Temple. There were compelling reasons against all of these.

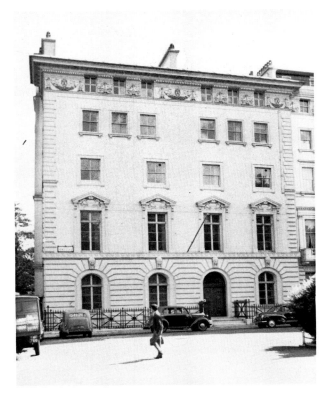

Plate 15 14 Princes Gate, London SW7

It was Mrs Thelma Glyn Hughes, the wife of our Honorary Treasurer of Council, who found us 13–14 Princes Gate, London SW7. It had been previously, between the two World Wars, the residence of the American Ambassador to the Court of St James's. Some of the Kennedy family had been brought up there in the late 1930s. The two houses No 13 and 14 had been cleverly joined together by Mr Pierpont Morgan to make one very pleasant large building with more than 50 rooms. It overlooked Hyde Park to the north and Ennismore Gardens to the south, with a large and attractive raised garden-balcony with shrubs and flowers.

It had been on the market for only a very short time; several people wanted it, including the Danish Embassy who, we were told, had cabled to Denmark for permission to buy it. We had to make a decision very quickly. I remember four of us meeting on the doorstep when we agreed to sign a cheque for £17 500 as a deposit, with an option to buy subject to a satisfactory surveyor's report and with the agreement of Council. Both

186

these came through satisfactorily. On July 26 1962 the contract was signed by the President of our College, George Abercrombie, and this magnificent, large double-fronted freehold building was ours. This was one of the most important incidents in our young College's life.

The price of the freehold was £175 000; alterations and redecorations added another £15 000 to the cost. It proved to be just what we wanted. Since then its value has increased greatly. We could hardly have made a better investment. The College owes an enormous debt to Mrs Thelma Glyn Hughes for the essential part she played in finding this splendid house for us. In 1962 we made her an Honorary Fellow of our College.

The move from 41 Cadogan Gardens to Princes Gate began on November 2 1962 – ten years after the College was founded. A sherry party was held there that evening. The offices and their staffs moved in on January 2 1963.

The building consisted of a large hall, with reception offices on the ground floor, a reception room (with a carpet made in Hong Kong depicting the College's Coat of Arms) opening on to the garden balcony, a dining

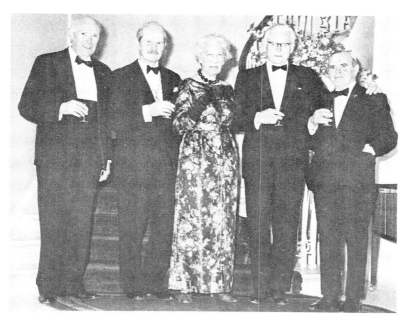

Plate 16 Five College Presidents on the stairs of 14 Princes Gate before a dinner in honour of John Hunt and the presentation to him of a silver salver engraved with the signatures of all members of the Foundation Council. (Left to right) George Abercrombie, Ian Watson, Annis Gillie, John Hunt, Fraser Rose.

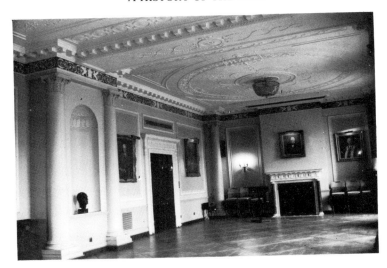

Plate 17   The Long Room

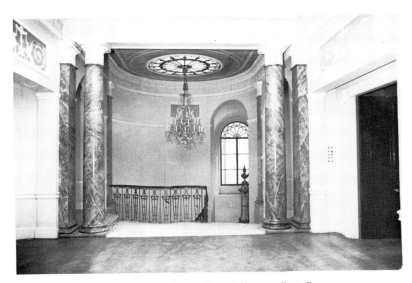

Plate 18   Interior of 14 Princes Gate. Chandelier on first floor

room and a fine curved staircase. On the first floor there was the 'Long Room' which held 100 people or more for dinners and lectures, a large quiet council room overlooking Ennismore Gardens; and the Geoffrey Evans

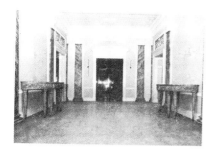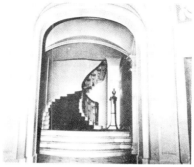

Plate 19   14 Princes Gate. Staircase and landing

Library with his portrait over the mantelpiece (see Chapter XIV). On the upper floors were offices, bedrooms, bathrooms etc, and in the basement, cloakrooms, a kitchen, a housekeeper's flat, more offices and storerooms.

By 1970 there was at Princes Gate a staff of 16. To a great many of them, who served us so well over the first 18 years, we owe our most grateful thanks. We cannot mention all their names here – Dr Sylvia Chapman, Commander A. E. P. Doran, Mrs Eileen Phillips, Miss Margaret Hammond, Mrs Joan Mant, Elizabeth Petrie (now Mrs Oliver Jayne), Mrs Hilda Larrington, Mrs B. Davey, Mrs Janet Bolton (now Mrs Smith, who has typed most of this book in her spare time) Mr C. V. Rees and Mrs Ada Fishley. And we must not forget all those who have done so much for the Scottish and other regional councils and faculties, at home and abroad, as well as all those in our research and educational organizations outside London.

In December 1970 James Wood joined the College as Administrative Secretary, in succession to Eileen Phillips. His responsibility was to provide an efficient and economical administration, capable of lightening the load which had been borne for so long on the shoulders of the officers and members of Council and its committees. It is interesting to consider how much and how quickly the College was still growing at that time. The total membership in June 1970 was 7416. In June 1977 after the formation of other organizations concerned with general practice in other countries such as Australia, New Zealand, South Africa, Malaysia and Singapore (leading to a decrease in the number of our overseas members), the total was 7991. The number sitting the membership examinations in November 1969 and May 1970 was 94; the corresponding figure in 1977 was 828. Expenditure in 1970 was £63 000; in 1977 it was £210 000. The total number of staff employed at headquarters (excluding domestic) in 1970 was 16; in 1977 it was 26, including the staff partly or wholly employed on the work of the Joint Committee on Postgraduate Training for General Practice and the Central Information Service, both of which were serviced by the College.

The 1970s saw a gradual shift on to the lay staff of much of the work hitherto undertaken by the honorary officers of Council and its committees. It also saw a strengthening of that staff, so that it could reflect adequately the increasing importance of the work which the College was doing. For example, in 1970 there was no full-time secretariat at Princes Gate for research, for practice organization or for the membership examination. The whole of undergraduate, postgraduate and continuing education was serviced by one secretary. The bulk of the work in all these fields fell, at that time, on to the shoulders of the chairmen and honorary secretaries of the various committees.

The administration of the College was therefore developed to reflect its activities, to serve them and to assist in their expansion. The framework of this administrative organization already existed: a small central secretariat servicing the Council itself and departments responsible for the work of each of the main activities of the College – the Board of Censors, Education, Research, the Examination and Practice Organization. To these must be added the work of the Finance Committee, the Investment Committee, the Registry, Publications, the Library, the *Journal* Office, and a supportive role for the Print Room, the Accommodation Secretary and the domestic staff. The purpose of this organization was to serve the College as a whole – its Council, central committees, regional faculties and its individual fellows, members and associates.

One important step in this development was the appointment of a Dean of Studies in 1974. Not only did he bring together various strands of medical education for general practice, but he was able to assist in the work of the college tutors appointed to the Postgraduate Medical Centres and to organize visits to training practices and the approval of Vocational Training Schemes. Without this medical presence in the administration of vocational training, the work of the Joint Committee on Postgraduate Training could not easily have achieved fruition. John Horder was the first Dean of Studies, assisted and eventually succeeded by Jack Norell.

As the College's views were increasingly sought by official bodies and its support canvassed for many causes, demand on its administrative staff increased. In an effort to contain the numbers of staff as the flood of paperwork surged on, the College enlisted the help of computers and word-processors in the administration of its affairs – first with the direct-debit method of collecting subscriptions in 1974 (itself a considerable saving in staff), then the distribution of the *Journal*, and latterly with the organization of the membership examination. This early mechanisation of routine work resulted in an improved ability to analyse and assist in forecasting trends and in helping to make decisions. Its further development will provide an essential administrative tool for storage and speedy recall of information, increasingly required in serving the complex web of College activities.

15 PRINCES GATE

In the summer of 1975 the College was approached by the owner of 15 Princes Gate, the house next door, who wished to sell it. He was asking £500 000, which was beyond our means. For family reasons the owner wished to retain the ground and first floor flats for his own use for a maximum of 12 years. This proviso made the property unattractive to most other potential buyers. A year later the College was able to negotiate a more favourable purchase price – £323 000 – of which an initial payment of £143 000 needed to be made at once, the remainder (interest-free) in 12 equal annual instalments of £15 000 each.

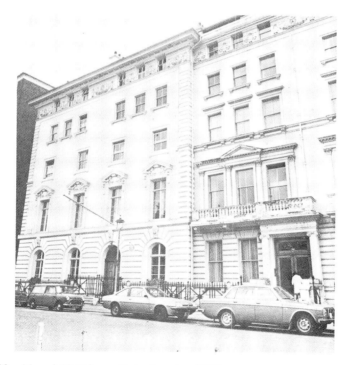

Plate 20   14 and 15 Princes Gate, London SW7

Throughout these negotiations the College's Investment Committee, on which sat distinguished financiers, was consulted and expressed its full agreement with the deal. The College's surveyors had previously indicated that extensive repairs to the fabric would be necessary and the opportunity was taken of putting in a new central heating system to meet the needs of the whole of the headquarters.

In December 1976, the College completed negotiations for this neighbouring house to provide more accommodation for members and associates and greatly needed additional office space. It contained six flats, with the owner, Mr Senley, occupying a maisonette on the ground and first floors. The terms of the agreement gave the College a 950-year lease of the building, with the owner retaining occupancy of his maisonette for 12 years from 1976. At the end of that time, or if he decided to move out earlier, the College had the option to purchase his part.

Much construction work had to be undertaken to convert the existing flats in this third house to offices and bedroom accommodation and to make communicating doors. Much of the furnishing and decoration was donated by regional councils and faculties.

At the end of its first 25 years the College administration had to meet the needs of a membership and associateship rapidly approaching 9000 general practitioners and steadily increasing each year. In addition it was beginning to serve the whole of general practice in the British Isles in various ways, through the work of the Joint Committee on Postgraduate Training, the Central Information Service and the Library. Another significant development was the increasing need for helping research and educational activities in Europe and closer ties with medical colleagues looking to us for a lead. Although this had occurred, to some extent, in many parts of the world since the birth of the College more than 25 years ago, our entry into the European Economic Community heralded new responsibilities for the future.

XVI
COLLEGE FINANCE AND APPEAL

Stuart J. Carne and Ancrum Evans (College Auditor)

COLLEGE FINANCE

The Royal College of General Practitioners was founded as an act of faith. The Steering Committee made a prophetic forecast:

> As the College grows, sufficient funds will be forthcoming if its work proves to be good and useful.

The secretarial expenses of the Steering Committee were met out of gifts for this purpose.

The members of the Finance and General Purposes Committee of the first College Council were G. F. Abercrombie (Chairman), F. M. Rose (Vice-Chairman), H. L. Glyn Hughes (Honorary Treasurer) and J. H. Hunt (Honorary Secretary). The Committee met 11 times during 1954.

With the increase in size and the activities of the College expenditure rose.

It was agreed that an allocation of up to ten shillings a year per member and associate of the faculty would be a fair method of distributing monies to each faculty. For overseas faculties, the yearly allocation would be equal to half the annual subscription of the members and associates.

Foundation members (those joining the original College between November 19 1952 and November 14 1953, the date of the first Annual General Meeting) paid an entrance fee of ten guineas.

The original financial policy of the College was that half the subscriptions from foundation members should be taken to capital and kept intact, and that the remainder should be allocated to expenditure over the first two years. [Financial Report 1955]

After allocating the appropriate amount for expenditure, a Founders' Capital Account of £14586 was established.

Annual subscriptions (initially three guineas per annum) were introduced on July 1 1954. It was hoped that these subscriptions would meet the running costs of the College. Therefore the entrance fee (ten guineas per member) was set to a Capital Reserve which, by March 31 1961 totalled £19909. The subscription income was adequate for the financial year ending June 30 1955 but for many years thereafter expenditure exceeded income. Between July 1 1955 and March 31 1961, when the College was incorporated as a company, the accumulated deficit rose to £14606. This debt was wiped off against the capital reserve fund leaving a credit balance of £5303. This was added to the original Founders' Capital Account, giving the new Incorporated College a new Founders' Capital Account of £19889, at which level it stayed for 25 years.

The Incorporated College thus began its life on April 1 1961 without a capital reserve. That year the practice of crediting the whole of the entrance fees to the capital reserve was continued but for the decade between 1962 and 1972 these fees, together with the fellowship enrolment fees and life subscriptions (an option open to members who had retired from practice) were divided equally between the capital reserve and the income and expenditure account. In 1972 the Capital Reserve had reached £32990 and College Council decided that no further monies needed to be put aside for this purpose. Subsequently all these sources of revenue have been allocated to income.

Fellows were elected for the first time in 1967. Their original enrolment fee was 25 guineas (reduced in appropriate circumstances to 15 guineas, or waived). Fellows paid the same annual subscriptions as members.

Foundation associates paid an entrance fee of one guinea but, like the foundation members, they paid no annual subscription until July 1954, when a subcription of one guinea a year was introduced and the entrance fee for associates temporarily abolished. Their annual subscription was doubled four years later and subsequently it has been increased in set stages. Since 1971 it has been set at parity with that for members. An entrance fee for associates was reintroduced in 1966.

The normal annual subscription for members was raised in 1959 from three to five guineas, in spite of which expenditure continued to exceed income, and by an increasing amount each year. By March 31 1966 the accumulated deficit of the College totalled £84000.

Administrative problems arose. Council (on the advice of its Finance and General Purposes Committee) asked Cooper Brothers (Consultant Accountants) to report. One of their many recommendations was that a separate Finance Committee be formed.

The original Finance and General Purposes Committee of Council held its first meeting on January 21 1953. H.L. Glyn Hughes joined it in February and was elected honorary treasurer on April 15. A separate Finance Committee was formed in January 1955. It met eight times, but in December of that year it was reunited with the General Purposes Committee.

Dr Glyn Hughes remained in office as honorary treasurer until November 1964. He had a very distinguished First and Second World War record, ending with the substantive rank of Brigadier and being awarded, after the Battle of Arnhem, a third Bar to the DSOs he had received in the 1914–18 war. He was also awarded a CBE for his services as DDMS Second Army. Perhaps his most distinguished activity was when he was Senior Medical Officer in the sector of the British Army of the Rhine which liberated some of the infamous Nazi concentration camps, including Belsen. His efforts led to the saving of many thousands of lives. His name was, and still is, held in the greatest respect by the survivors of that camp.

Between the wars he was a general practitioner on Dartmoor and later in London. After the war he entered medical administration and was the first Senior Administrative Medical Officer of the South-east London Regional Hospital Board. Though compulsorily retired from that job by age, he remained active and played a major role in the opening of the Peckham (General Practice) Centre.

Outside medicine he was also internationally known for his skill on the rugby football field and as President of the Barbarians' Rugby Club.

He died in November 1973 and his Thanksgiving Service held in St Marylebone Parish Church was filled with eminent men and women from all walks of life – the Army, sport, the ranks of those who had suffered in the concentration camps, and from all branches of medicine including leading members of our own College. He had requested that all those who attended his Thanksgiving Service should wear 'Club' ties.

A new Finance Committee of the College was formed in 1964, with Stuart Carne succeeding Glyn Hughes as honorary treasurer. Its terms of reference were:

To consider all matters connected with the finances of the College, to advise Council on all financial matters and to take executive action on Council's financial policy.

The first aim of the new Finance Committee was to control the College expenditure and this it did, with the effect that, in its first year, the College deficit, for the first time since 1956, did not rise above the previous year's level. However, it was necessary to make the College solvent. It could have been done by reducing to a bare minimum all college activities. This, in the opinion of the Finance Committee, would have impeded the development of the College.

All possible ways of dealing with the deficit were considered and most were rejected. The Finance Committee believed that the members would be willing to support *their* College and so, at the 1965 Annual General Meeting they proposed that the annual subscription be doubled from five to ten guineas. An application fee of £21 was introduced and the entrance fee was raised to £15.

As a result of the increase in the members' subscriptions, the College income exceeded its expenditure every year since 1967 except for the two years 1972/73 and 1973/74. In 1975/76 a deficit almost occurred, but it was proposed at the Annual General Meeting that members be invited to pay an additional voluntary subscription pending the introduction of a new rate. £16 000 was raised and a record potential deficit of £11 000 was converted into a surplus of £5000.

At its height, at the end of the 1965/66 financial year, before the doubled subscription came into effect, the accumulated deficit stood at £84 000. Among its debtors was the College Appeal, from the capital of which £37 000 had been borrowed in the late 1950s and early 1960s. At the Annual General Meeting it was agreed that in future the College would not use appeal money for this purpose.

The accumulated deficit was finally cleared in 1971. For the first time since the foundation of the College, the accumulated funds stood in credit. By then, however, inflation was beginning to be strongly felt. Our total income that year was £73 982 (of which £63 822 came from annual subscriptions). Two years later our income was just short of £100 000 and only four years after that, in 1976/77 it exceeded £200 000. Part of this, of course, reflected expansion of the College's activities, outlined in other chapters of this book.

THE APPEAL

In 1959 it was apparent that if the progress of the College, in its various spheres of activity, was to be maintained an appeal to the general public had become a necessity. The first Appeal Committee was formed in 1959 with H. L. Glyn Hughes as Chairman and R. Cove-Smith as honorary secretary. In planning and launching this appeal the College received invaluable advice and assistance from Sir Harry Jephcott, chairman of Glaxo Ltd, whose generous and magnificent efforts over the next few years were largely responsible for the excellent results.

A brochure was prepared which outlined the ideals of the College and the aims and objects of the Appeal. A charming foreword was written for this by Sir Arthur Bryant.

The objective of the Appeal was to raise money for the following purposes:

(1) *To build and equip a permanent home.*
College headquarters in Cadogan Gardens at that time was held on a lease, and it was already evident that with the increasing work and stature of the College a larger and permanent home would become a necessity in the near future.

(2) *To establish a research foundation.*
Research was a major activity of the College at all levels. It was progressing rapidly but without adequate finances was bound to be retarded.

(3) *To develop the College's educational activities, both undergraduate and postgraduate.*
Much had already been done in the field of education, but development could not proceed without additional financial help.

The Appeal began by an approach to all members and associates, and by the personal help of the sponsors and others. It was launched publicly on March 4 1960. By the end of that year a sum of £330 000 had been received.

The first approaches all emanated from College headquarters, but it was proposed to make a second major effort in October 1960 and in this phase to rely very largely on the faculties throughout the country who, with their local knowledge and close association with the community, would follow up some approaches and initiate others.

Trustees appointed under the chairmanship of Sir Harry Jephcott included Lord Nathan and Lord Cohen of Birkenhead, together with representatives of the College Council and its Research Committee.

By 1962 the total figure had reached £381 766, of which members and associates had contributed £35 941.

The purchase of the freehold of 14 Princes Gate absorbed a considerable proportion of the capital monies and the establishment of the Research Foundation Board had further depleted the total (see Chapter XI).

Faculties were stimulated to play their full part and many of them responded admirably and achieved encouraging results. They were given complete freedom to approach local firms and organizations in their areas.

During 1970 a lay committee was formed to assist the Appeal Committee in making a fresh approach to industry. The members were: Mr Ellis Stanning, Sir Arthur Smith, Mr Hilton Clark, Sir George Pope and Mr E. Guiseppi, to whom the College was most grateful for all the help they gave.

Appeal money was given to the College Foundations (Research, Education and Medical Recording Service) and to the Headquarters and General Endowment Fund. It was also used to maintain the structure of College headquarters and other buildings. No money from the appeal fund was put towards the day-to-day expenses.

By then £475 911 had been promised, of which £443 900 had already been received and the rest was due under covenant. Of these donations, £60 000 had been given or promised under covenant by 110 members and associates of the College. The fact that they had given so much over and above their annual subscriptions was an indication of the worth they placed upon the College.

A further Appeal was launched in June 1972. A special effort by Welsh Council began with a ceremony in July; in the October the West of Scotland faculty raised over £840 at a dinner and dance and other fund-raising activities; the Yorkshire faculty held a Press Conference in the November; and in May 1973 a generous contribution was made by members living in Northern Ireland. Scottish Council set up an appeal subcommittee to encourage and assist individual initiative by members in bringing the work of the College to the notice of their friends and patients, especially those connected with industry.

Well over 100 companies and organizations made covenants or donations totalling approximately £94 000 (see 1973 *Annual Report*, page 50). Every one of these was the result of a personal approach by a sponsor or member of the College. Our sponsors reminded us repeatedly that the money and the goodwill was there, but our members themselves had to take the initiative in approaching people in their own practices and locality, inviting their practical support for the future work of the College. By 1977, when the College was 25 years old, the Appeal had raised £619 343.

XVII
AWARDS AND ETHICAL COMMITTEES

Annis C. Gillie, John H. Hunt and Basil C. S. Slater

AWARDS COMMITTEE

AWARDS COMMITTEE

The Awards Committee (with G. F. Abercrombie as Chairman and J. H. Hunt as honorary Secretary) in 1955 recommended to Council that the Foundation Council Award – a legacy from the members of the Foundation Council of the College, to be given occasionally and only 'for work of the highest merit in the realm of general practice or for service of the greatest distinction to the cause of general practice' – be presented to R. J. Minnitt of Liverpool. At the Annual General Meeting, the President handed to him a miniature replica, in silver mounted on ebony, of the gavel presented to the College by His Excellency the Greek Ambassador, M. Basile Mostras, in 1953.

The committee considered 12 essays on 'The Influence of Home Conditions during the First Five Years of Life on the Physical and Mental Health of Children' and recommended that the Butterworth Gold Medal presented for the first time in 1955 be awarded to D. W. MacLean, a Foundation Associate, of the General Practice Teaching Unit, University of Edinburgh.

The committee recommended to Council that:

(1) The initials MCGP should not be used after names at present.

(2) Six names, already agreed, namely the chairman and consultant members of the Steering Committee – The Rt Hon Henry Willink, QC, Professor Ian Aird, Mr John Beattie, Sir Wilson Jameson, Professor J. M. Mackintosh and Sir Heneage Ogilvie – be put

forward that year for election by the College to Honorary Fellowship.

(3) A grade of Fellowship be established.

(4) A Fellowship should only be awarded to members of at least five years' standing, who had rendered special service to general practice and/or to the College.

(5) The award of Fellowship should be strictly limited.

For the names of further Honorary Fellows and winners of medals and prizes readers should consult Appendix 1 and the *Annual Reports*.

At its meeting in December 1956, the committee agreed that its terms of reference be amended to read:

To advise and assist Council on all questions of awards, lecture-ships, honours, regalia and ceremonies.

In 1957, at the request of Benger Laboratories Ltd, who had most generously contributed 250 guineas for the general purposes of the College, the awards committee studied 88 entries for the competition on 'Original Observations in General Practice' and selected the three prizewinners.

A design for a presidential chain was approved by Council and made to the order of Geigy Pharmaceutical Company Ltd, to whom the College was very deeply indebted for the most handsome and original gift (see Chapter XIX).

In 1960 Annis Gillie was in consultation with Mr James Laver on the subject of academic dress (see Chapter XIX) and with Lord Amulree on the project for fixing a plaque on 17 Bentinck Street, London, to commemorate Sir James Mackenzie's residence there.

Council was invited to propose two names to the trustees of the James Mackenzie Prize. It was awarded for the first time in 1961 to G. I. Watson. This substantial monetary prize (approximately £1000) was to be given every five years to a general practitioner in the British Commonwealth who had published or undertaken some valuable work during that period.

A new attendance book, bound in leather and embossed on the outside, was presented to the Council of the incorporated College 'to commemorate the work of the Steering Committee'. The College's achievement of arms was finally settled (see Chapter XIX).

In 1962 Geigy Pharmaceutical Company Ltd offered to present a pendant to complete the presidential chain of office and this offer was gratefully accepted. A smaller design was approved for use as a badge for provosts (see Chapter XIX).

In 1963 Council invited the Rt Reverend George E. Reindorp, Bishop of Guildford, to become honorary chaplain of the College.

A corporate seal had been struck for the sealing of official college documents.

ETHICAL COMMITTEE

The Ethical Committee was formed in 1960, with Annis Gillie as chairman and G. I. Watson as honorary secretary. This subcommittee of the Finance and General Purposes Committee was formed

> To advise and assist the Finance and General Purposes Committee
> of Council on all ethical matters connected with college activities.

It met on several occasions during its first year and gave particular attention to drafting a code for the use of the College, centrally and at faculty level, for relationships with pharmaceutical and other business houses.

Other problems were discussed, particularly that of the ethical issues raised by controlled trials of vaccine therapy.

The following year it became a full committee of College Council with G. I. Watson as chairman and J. M. Henderson as honorary secretary. (For officers and members of the committee during the following years, see the *Annual Reports*). This full committee drew up and circulated an ethical code, relating particularly to all offers of gifts or financial assistance made on behalf of the College to individuals, faculty boards, committees of Council or to officers of Council. Two of the principal recommendations accepted by Council were:

(1) In future the name of a commercial firm (whether pharmaceutical or otherwise) should not be attached to any new award, prize, lecture, scholarship or research programme accepted by the College; but there was no objection, in principle, to linking the name of any doctor, distinguished non-medical person, or benefactor of the College, with the title of an award, provided that prior approval of Council had been obtained.

(2) The normal form of acknowledgement of gifts, apart from an immediate letter, should be a statement of appreciation in the Annual Report, and only in exceptional circumstances should any other form of acknowledgement be authorized by Council.

Council also accepted the committee's advice about the need for prior consultation with Council or its officers before gifts or other assistance was accepted on behalf of the College, including the holding of College symposia, and other matters concerning the good name of the College.

In 1964 the committee recommended to Council that, if the General Medical Council were to remove the name of a doctor from the Medical Register, that doctor's link with the College would automaticaly be broken, but in the committee's view the College would be unwise to censure any member or associate under any circumstances that could not be foreseen.

The committee discussed some of the ethical difficulties which would arise when the promoters of a training course for laymen or women sought the help of members or faculties of the College in showing their students general practice 'from the inside', either in a surgery or on a round of visits. In its view:

(1) There was no fundamental ethical objection to general practioners helping with the training of students so long as each doctor came to his own independent decision about accepting such trainees in his practice.

(2) Each patient, particularly in surgery sessions, should be asked if he had any objection to the presence of such a student, without the trainee being present when the question was put.

(3) A distinction should be drawn between help with the training of medical or nursing students or recognized medical auxiliaries and with that of others whose qualifications (if any) were not recognized.

(4) It was unethical to take a student further into the details of any patient's case than was strictly necessary for the student's training.

In 1965 the committee recommended that, since the College Register was not published or offered for sale outside the College, members of the public should not be provided with copies, for use as a mailing list or similar purpose. The Research Committee had always taken this view about the Research Register and Council agreed that this precedent should be followed.

THE AWARDS AND ETHICAL COMMITTEE

In 1966 the Awards and Ethical Committees were combined into one committee of Council with terms of reference:

To assist Council on all questions of awards, lectureships, honours, insignia and ceremonies.

In 1968 these were changed to:

> To advise and assist Council on all questions of awards, lecture-
> ships, honours, insignia and ceremonies, and on all ethical matters
> concerning the College.

The Education Foundation had endowed an annual William Pickles
Lecture to be delivered at the spring general meetings of the College, and
the first was delivered by P. S. Byrne in 1968. (For other William Pickles
Lecturers, see Appendix 6.)

In 1970 Council accepted the committee's advice that an award, to be
called the George Abercrombie Award, should be given for outstanding
contributions to the literature of general practice, and agreed that the first
recipient of this award should be R. M. S. McConaghey. (For other
recipients, see Appendix 8.)

Certificates for fellowship and membership were agreed and printed in
that year.

At the Annual General Meeting in 1972 HRH The Prince Philip, Duke
of Edinburgh, was appointed an Honorary Fellow of the College before
being elected President.

In 1974 the British Migraine Association made available three prizes
entitled the 'Migraine Trust Prize' to be awarded by the College on 'The
Natural History of Migraine and its Management in General Practice'. The
competition was open only to trainees in general practice on vocational
training schemes or undergoing a one-year traineeship in general practice.

XVIII
INCORPORATION, ROYAL PREFIX AND THE
ROYAL CHARTER

John Mayo

The plans for the incorporation of the College and its ultimate transition to a Royal College incorporated by Royal Charter were laid by the Steering Committee at its fifth meeting held on September 17 1952. This followed a report by John Mayo, our College Solicitor, of Messrs Linklater and Paines on a visit by his senior partner, Sir Sam Brown, and himself to the (then) Board of Trade where they had discussed the formation of the College with Mr J. Cowen (Assistant Secretary of the Insurance and Companies Department) and a colleague, Mr I. de Keyser, who came from a medical family and advised him on medical matters. Sir Sam Brown had been introduced to John Hunt by a friend and patient of his, Henry Benson (later Lord Benson) of Cooper Brothers (accountants) to whom the College owes a considerable debt of gratitude.

At the Steering Committee meeting I ruled out the possibility of a Royal College at the outset. I advised on following the conventional route of starting as a company limited by guarantee with a name excluding the word 'Limited' by licence of the Board of Trade under Section 19 of the Companies Act 1948 relating to associations to be formed for promoting commerce, art, science, religion, charity or any other useful object. I explained the procedures to be followed, including the fact that the Board of Trade would seek advice on the application from established institutions in the medical field. Mr Cowen had indicated that the Board of Trade would probably refer to the Principal Medical Officer of the Ministry of Health, the British Medical Association, the three (then-existing) medical

Royal Colleges in London and possibly the British Postgraduate Medical Federation of the University of London. At the best, if there was no opposition at all, the application would not go through in less than four to six months and, if there was any opposition from any of the referees, the application might take a couple of years and at the end could be turned down. As the Steering Committee felt that there would be a considerable measure of opposition to the establishment of the new College, the idea of a Section 19 application did not seem very attractive.

To get a Section 19 licence would, however, be a much easier and more satisfactory proposition once the College had been formed and had proved its worth and established good relations with other medical bodies. It was therefore suggested to the Steering Committee that a convenient and suitable way to proceed would be to start off as an unincorporated association (akin to a club) with a view to applying, later, for incorporation and a Royal Charter. The legal suggestion was to set up the College with an interim constitution in the form of Memorandum and Articles of Association nearly the same as those appropriate for incorporation, so that very little change would be needed when the College moved to incorporation. To be as certain as possible that the interim constitution would go through the Board of Trade in due course as a final constitution with minimum change, I suggested having the draft cleared by Mr Cecil Turner, a senior company barrister to whom the Board of Trade customarily submitted for approval the proposed Memorandum and Articles of Association put forward by any applicant for a Section 19 licence. The Board of Trade had indicated that there was no objection to Mr Cecil Turner advising individual clients on such matters.

In response to a question as to how long might elapse after setting up as an unincorporated College and before applying for incorporation, the answer was that it would have to be at least a year and perhaps several years and that it would be unwise to rush on to the next stage. An established financial position or strong financial backing was of importance in the view of the Board of Trade.

So far as is known no unincorporated association had previously been established with a Memorandum and Articles of Association – indeed it is probable that down to the present day there has been no other example. The drafting was nevertheless completed within a few days and, after the draft had been gone through with John Hunt, a proof print was prepared dated 3 October 1952 and submitted to Mr Cecil Turner for approval. The opening paragraphs of the Instructions to Counsel set out the objective and longer-term plans of the Steering Committee. They were:

The College of General Practitioners is intended to carry out in respect of general medical practitioners functions corresponding to those carried out by The Royal College of Physicians, The Royal College of Surgeons and The Royal College of Obstetricians and Gynaecologists in relation to their respective members. It is somewhat surprising that such a body was not formed many years ago and in fact over 100 years ago a proposal to form such a body did reach the stage of a draft Act of Parliament which was however never passed [see Chapter I]. During the last few years there has been active correspondence on the matter and at the beginning of this year a Steering Committee was formed under the chairmanship of The Rt Hon H. U. Willink, QC, Master of Magdalene College, Cambridge, and a former Minister of Health, with a view to the formation of such a body.

The Steering Committee has decided that in the first instance an unincorporated association should be formed under the name of The College of General Practitioners of the United Kingdom* with the intention that at a later date application will be made for the incorporation of a company limited by guarantee under the same name with the licence of the Board of Trade under section 19 of the Companies Act, 1948. At a still later stage it is hoped that a Royal Charter will be granted.

It is desired that the constitution of the unincorporated association should be as nearly as possible the same as that which would be required upon the formation of a company limited by guarantee and accordingly a draft constitution has been prepared in the form of a Memorandum and Articles of Association.

It is desired that the College shall rank for tax purposes as a charity and the objects of the College have been drafted on this basis. It may be however that with this in mind the objects have been somewhat narrowly framed. If Counsel is of the opinion that the powers of the College under the existing draft are likely to be insufficient Counsel is requested to consider whether the objects can be amended so as to give somewhat wider powers to the College without affecting its charitable status.

The draft Memorandum and Articles of Association were settled by Counsel, who gave a covering Opinion dated 30 October 1952 indicating that, subject to any change in the policy of the Board of Trade regarding questions of practice and principle, no material changes would be likely to

---

* The words 'of the United Kingdom' represented an idea of a member of the Steering Committee but the words were later considered and rejected by the Steering Committee.

be required by the Board of Trade when incorporation was sought. On 19 November 1952 at its eighth and final meeting the General Practice Steering Committee approved, completed the signature of and dated the Memorandum and Articles of Association by the ten General Practitioner members of the Committee (thus formally constituting the College) and at the same time approved and signed its Report entitled 'A College of General Practitioners' which was to appear in the *British Medical Journal* (No. 4798, p. 1321) on 20 December 1952, courtesy letters of notification having been sent to over 400 people, including in particular the Presidents of the Royal Colleges, the Secretary of the British Medical Association, the Secretaries of its Divisions, the Deans of the Medical Schools and the medical Members of Parliament.

The Steering Committee's Report summarized the plans for the constitutional future of the College in these brief terms:

> At first it is intended that the college shall operate as an unincorp- orated association: in a few years' time we hope that it will have proved its worth sufficiently to justify application for incorporation under the same name, and later for a Royal Charter.

The 'few years' envisaged by the Steering Committee may appear to have been an underestimate, but this is not really so. The period which elapsed before incorporation was not so much because the College did not progress as envisaged, but because it was generally felt that incorporation could best wait until one could be totally confident both that the College would have the support of all the other medical bodies and that the requirements of the Board of Trade (later Department of Trade) would un- questionably be met.

The relevant requirements of the Board of Trade were those in relation to the granting of a licence under section 19 of the Companies Act 1948 to permit a body to become incorporated with limited liability but without the word 'Limited' having to appear at the end of its name. Section 19 is available in the case of an association about to be formed as a limited company for the purpose of promoting commerce, art, science, religion, charity or any other useful object, which intends to apply its profits (if any) or other income to promoting its objects and to prohibit the division of any such profit among its members. As has earlier been stated the original College constitution was formed so as to require minimum alteration when the College moved to incorporation with a section 19 licence. Only in very special circumstances would the Board of Trade consider an application by a body not in a position to show by means of its past history that it had established itself as a body capable of carrying out the objects for which it was formed. That criterion the College was in a position to meet within a few years of its establishment. The other major criterion was that in all cases the Board of Trade must be satisfied that the financial position is secure.

The development of the financial position of the College can be seen from the figures extracted from the first ten yearly Financial Reports and Accounts and shown in Table 1.

Table 1.   The College's finances: first ten years

Financial year	Income £	Expenditure £	Net assets £
Period ended 30 June			
1953	2 507	2 030	17 713
1954	7 365	6 474	20 491
1955	9 419	7 845	22 317
1956	10 134	10 793	24 201
1957	11 237	14 279	24 239
1958	12 548	15 771	23 688
1959*	14 277	17 271	21 722
1960†	20 549	21 577	71 939
Period ended 31 March			
1961 (9 months)	15 960	20 887	104 198‡
1962	22 854	27 406	163 850§

It will be seen that from 1956 onwards the College was consistently producing an excess of expenditure over income. Even though these deficits represented in part the treatment of Entrance Fees as capital receipts, net assets were modest in amount and it was difficult to treat the financial position of the College as fully secure. In these circumstances, and since the College was operating satisfactorily in unincorporated form, the Council deemed an application for incorporation to be premature. The launching of the College Appeal in January 1960, transformed the financial situation. At 30 June 1960, the College Appeal (after deducting expenses) stood at £311 320 (including promised future payments of £258 613) with the result that (including promised future payments) the net assets of the College had multiplied nearly 16 times and (excluding promised future payments) had

* £2200 transferred to new Australian College of General Practitioners.
† College Appeal launched. Fund stands at £311 320 including covenanted future income of £258 613 not included in net assets.
‡ Covenanted future Appeal income of £259 271 not included in net assets.
§ Covenanted future Appeal income of £233 659 not included in net assets.

more than trebled. It is not surprising that in the year 1960 the Council was able to conclude that the financial position could be demonstrated to the Board of Trade as fully secure and that the time had come to apply for incorporation.

When application was made to the Board of Trade for a section 19 licence to permit incorporation as a limited company but omitting 'Limited' from the name, no problems were experienced and the original drafting of the Memorandum and Articles of Association in 1952 proved itself, since the changes needed for the purposes of the incorporated College were little more than the minimum essential as a matter of form. A new College in incorporated form was established on 8 February 1961.

The unincorporated College and the new incorporated College existed side by side for a while. By the combined result of a provision in the Articles of Association of the new College and of a Special Resolution passed by the members of the old College, all the persons who on 8 February 1961 were fellows, members or associates of the old College became entitled, on lodgement of written consent, to be fellows, members or associates of the incorporated College. In return for this privilege the new College became a member of the old College and all the other members vacated membership. In the result all the assets of the old College became owned by the new College. The old College was, nevertheless, kept in existence for some years, because it (rather than the new College) was the beneficiary of a number of deeds of covenant given by donors to the College Appeal and it was desirable to avoid any technical legal hiatus, even though it would probably never have been noticed.

THE ROYAL PREFIX

The Steering Committee and the Foundation Council had envisaged that the College would become a Royal College at the stage when a Royal Charter was obtained. The event differed from the expectation.

Early in 1967 the President (then Dame Annis Gillie) wrote to Rear-Admiral C. Bonham-Carter in pursuance of his offer to approach His Royal Highness The Prince Philip, Duke of Edinburgh, with regard to Royal Patronage of the College. Prince Philip was good enough to state that he was much in favour of having a connection with the College but he suggested that the College would get more out of him [!] if the connection was formed as part of some special anniversary year and offered to be President for the twentieth or twenty-first Anniversary year (1972 or 1973). Needless to say that suggestion was greeted with acclaim and the College had to consider how to adjust the Constitution to permit his appointment

210

since, although he had acted at one time in his professional life as a 'doctor' in a small ship, the lawyers had tied up the constitution tiresomely to registered medical practitioners only. As we shall later see, such a problem is easily overcome.

In April 1967 an official in the Home Office wrote in the following terms:

> I have the honour, by direction of the Home Secretary, to inform you that The Queen has been graciously pleased to command that the College of General Practitioners shall, in future, be known as the Royal College of General Practitioners.

The College acted in accordance with the command of Her Majesty and the writing paper was changed forthwith. What had escaped our notice was that since the College was a company incorporated by statute it was able to change its name only in the manner provided by the statute. Some few months went by before the College Solicitor spotted the position and drew attention to the need to change the name of the College in the manner provided by law!

Although Her Majesty had agreed to the change of name, it was necessary to go through the procedure in accordance with the provisions of the Companies Act 1948 and for this purpose a Board of Trade official, the Registrar of Companies, had to be requested to issue a consent. Fortunately the Board of Trade was willing to give this. The Agenda for the 1967 Annual General Meeting went out headed:

THE COLLEGE OF GENERAL PRACTITIONERS

(name about to be changed to

THE ROYAL COLLEGE OF GENERAL PRACTITIONERS

and on 17 November 1967, a Special Resolution was passed in the following terms:

> That in accordance with the wishes of Her Majesty The Queen the name of the College be changed to 'The Royal College of General Practitioners'.

Note: The actual date on which the change of name became effective was 6 December 1967, when a Certificate of Incorporation on Change of Name was issued by the Assistant Registrar of Companies.

THE ROYAL CHARTER

The grant of a Royal Charter is not easily obtained and the procedures to be gone through are liable to take anything from nine months upwards even in the most worthy and uncontroversial case. Therefore action commenced in 1971 with a view to obtaining a Royal Charter in time for the planned appointment of Prince Philip as President at the 1972 Annual General Meeting. At the Spring General Meeting small alterations were made to the Articles of Association so that Prince Philip could be appointed as an Honorary Fellow and so that an Honorary Fellow was eligible for appointment as President. To obtain a Royal Charter an enabling Resolution was needed from the College in General Meeting and this was dealt with at the 1971 Annual General Meeting, in case the 1972 Spring General Meeting might not allow sufficient time. On 20 November 1971 a Special Resolution was passed at the AGM approving a Petition to Her Majesty for the grant of a Royal Charter similar in substance to the existing Memorandum and Articles of Association. The Petition was lodged with the Privy Council Office and the Board of Trade notified of the action taken.

One matter which I had to consider was that as a matter of law the chartered College would be a legal entity separate and distinct from the College incorporated under the Companies Act and *prima facie* all the assets would need to be transferred to the chartered College and transfers would give rise to a liability to *ad valorem* stamp duty. The method used to avoid such stamp duty on the transfer of assets from the unincorporated College to the incorporated College would not work on a transfer from one incorporated body to another. However the legal grapevine brought to light an unpublished statutory concession which operated for an incorporated charity moving to chartered status.

The Petition presented to Her Majesty in Council recited, in addition to the salient historical facts, a number of items of the then-current statistics, including the following:

(1) Since the establishment of the membership examination in 1968 there had been seven examinations with a total of 299 candidates (244 successful).

(2) At 20 November 1971 (the date of the AGM) there were 7567 fellows, members and associates.

(3) The College owned 14 Princes Gate (bookcost £195 415) and as at 31 March 1971 investments and monies on deposit of a total value of £335 118.

(4) In the year to 30 June 1971 admission fees received were £6287 and annual subscriptions £63 822.

The Petition ended with the words, 'AND YOUR PETITIONERS would ever pray etc'. The 'etc' was not a slip-up due to a typist failing to type in the intended standard wording. In fact the wording which originally followed the prayer became lost in history and for hundreds of years back petitioners have been driven to the use of 'et cetera'. We know not what we pray!

At the time of the lodgement of the Petition with the Privy Council Office a draft Charter and Ordinances were submitted for consideration and in parallel with the processing of the Petition (involving careful enquiries into the status and reputation of the College) the draft Charter and Ordinances were reviewed and some changes to these were discussed and agreed. One must feel some sympathy with the Privy Council Office in that, while the College's Petition had to be strictly considered in accordance with established criteria, the fact remained that any unfavourable conclusion or delay beyond the planned timetable would not have pleased Prince Philip. As, however, the College was wholly worthy, no problem arose in practice. The planned timetable had in fact to be accelerated a little as Prince Philip had to rearrange his appointments and accordingly requested a somewhat earlier date (1 November) for the Annual General Meeting than that (16 November) which he had earlier approved; plenty of notice of this change was given and the Privy Council Office was not therefore put in a position of difficulty. The grant of the Charter was approved at a Council held by Her Majesty The Queen on 23 October 1972 and (an £85 fee having been paid) the Charter was issued under the Great Seal on the following day. The Charter was formally handed over by His Royal Highness The Prince Philip, Duke of Edinburgh, on November 1 1972 at the Annual General Meeting, when he was appointed an Honorary Fellow and elected as President.

XIX
INSIGNIA AND THE COLLEGE GRACE

THE INSIGNIA

Dame Annis C. Gillie

The College Motto

From a very early stage in the development of the College the Council became aware of the need for a motto for the College aims with an obvious relation to the range of work of general practitioners. The consideration of this was begun by the first chairman of Council, G. F. Abercrombie, in his choice of a motto, brief but easily remembered by fellows, members and associates – the Latin phrase '*Cum Scientia Caritas*' was submitted to Council and unanimously agreed. Constant use of these words, with their contemporary English translation, for formal and informal occasions, has confirmed the wisdom of the choice. Many interpretations expressing the personal features of their work can be placed upon the phrase. They range from 'Skill with care' or 'Scientific knowledge applied with compassion' to the fuller one of 'Skill and scientific knowledge used with tender loving care', and others also.

Presidential Chain

In 1958 Geigy Pharmaceutical Company Ltd offered to meet the cost of a Presidential Chain. The matter was referred by Council to the Awards Committee, the chairman at that time being George Abercrombie. We conferred with Messrs Garrard and Company of London on the design of a chain 40 inches long. It was made by A. Styles, a member of the staff of

Garrards, in consultation with George Abercrombie. Links in white gold of a poppy intertwined with yellow gold foxgloves alternated with yellow gold links of twisted serpents. The craftsmanship was approved by the Design Research Centre of Great Britain. Council gave its approval and it was presented to the President at the Annual General Meeting of 1958.

The Presidential Badge and the College's Coat of Arms

The chain itself, though an admirable symbol of office, lacked a badge to hang from it. At that period the College had no coat of arms and the reponsibility for considering this was again passed to the Awards Committee. Discussions were long and many, when strong personal views were expressed.

It was agreed that the shield should be divided vertically into black and white halves suggestive of night and day, and a further division by a chevron, countercharged to suggest the roof of the house, in which most of general practice takes place. This left three places, two above and one below the dividing lines. The two above the chevron were charged with the white poppy indicating the relief of pain and suffering on the left, while on the right the gentian flower indicated the restorative and rehabilitating side of our work and provides a link with the coat of arms of Caius, as seen at the college named after him at Cambridge. The third space on the shield below the chevron is occupied by a Greek lamp to indicate the importance of study and of research in the work of the College, and its links with the lamp of nursing. Some discussion was caused by this; the alternative of an open volume was rejected on account of its limitations.

There was much dissension about the proposed supporters of the shield. The suggestion of two centaurs was discarded on the grounds of the confusing effect of six limbs apiece. A proposal to use the ox – the sign of St Luke, a reputed physician – as a supporter was opposed on the grounds that it was a primitively sacrificial animal. Finally, somewhat reluctant agreement was secured to the adoption of the unicorn from the Worshipful Society of Apothecaries on the dexter side, with the gold and silver reversed from that·of the royal unicorn, and the lynx from the arms of the Royal College of Surgeons. In spite of opposition from Ian Grant (then President) to 'that spotted cat!' we had, however, his final agreement. The generosity of the Worshipful Society of Apothecaries and the Royal College of Surgeons was duly acknowledged. The choice of the owl as the most ancient symbol of medicine, in chairman capacity with gavel entwined by serpent, provoked no opposition and, as the motto had been accepted earlier, there were no further delays. We owe much to the tolerance of the Colleges of

216

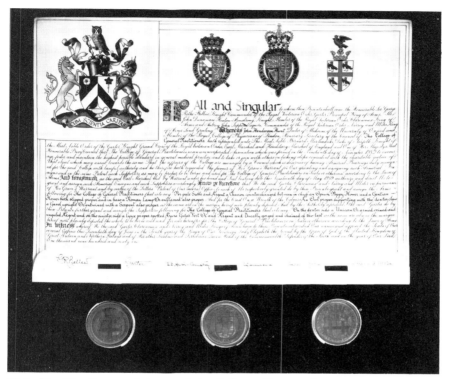

Plate 21   The Patent of Arms of the College. The text is:

TO ALL AND SINGULAR to whom the Presents shall come, the Honorable Sir George Rothe Bellew, Knight Commander of the Royal Victorian Order, Garter Principal King of Arms, Sir John Dunamace Heaton-Armstrong, Knight, Member of the Royal Victorian Order, Clarenceux King of Arms and Aubrey John Toppin, Esquire, Commander of the Royal Victorian Order, Norroy and Ulster King of Arms, Send Greeting! WHEREAS *John Henderson Hunt*, Doctor of Medicine of the University of Oxford and Member of the Royal College of Physicians of London, Honorary Secretary of the Council of *The College of General Practitioners*, hath represented unto The Most Noble Bernard Marmaduke, Duke of Norfolk, Knight of the Most Noble Order of the Garter, Knight Grand Cross of the Royal Victorian Order, Earl Marshal and Hereditary Marshal of England and One of Her Majesty's Most Honourable Privy Council, that The College of General Practitioners is an unincorporated Association which was formed on the Nineteenth day of November 1952 to encourage foster and maintain the highest possible standard in general medical practice and to take or join with others in taking steps consistent with the charitable nature of that object which may assist towards the same. That the affairs of the College are managed by a Council which is desirous of having Armorial Bearings duly assigned for the said College with lawful authority and he therefore hath requested the favour of His Grace's Warrant for Our granting and assigning such Armorial Ensigns and in the same Patent such Supporters as may be proper to be borne and used for The College of General Practitioners on Seals or otherwise according to the Laws of Arms AND FORASMUCH as the said Earl Marshal did by Warrant under his hand and Seal bearing date the Nineteenth day of May 1959 authorize and direct Us to grant and assign such Armorial Ensigns and such Supporters accordingly KNOW YE THEREFORE that We the said Garter Clarenceux and Norroy and Ulster in pursuance of His Grace's Warrant and by virtue of the Letters Patent of Our several offices to each of Us respectively granted do by these Presents grant and assign the Arms following for *The College of General Practitioners* that is to say:- *Per pale Sable and Argent a Chevron counterchanged between in chief an Opium Poppy Flower and a Gentian Flower both slipped proper and in base a Roman Lamp Or enflamed also proper* And for the Crest on a Wreath of the Colours *An Owl proper supporting with the dexter claw a Gavel upright Or entwined with a Serpent also proper* as the same are in the margin hereof more plainly depicted And by the Authority aforesaid I the said Garter do by these Presents further grant and assign the Supporters following for The College of General Practitioners that is to say:- *On the dexter side a Unicorn Or armed crined and unguled Argent and on the sinister side a Lynx proper spotted Azure Gules Vert Or and Argent and Ducally gorged and chained of the last* as the same are also in the margin hereof more plainly depicted the whole to be borne and used forever hereafter for The College of General Practitioners on Seals or otherwise according to the Laws of Arms. IN WITNESS whereof We the said Garter Clarenceux and Norroy and Ulster Kings of Arms have to these Presents subscribed Our names and affixed the Seals of Our several offices this Twentieth day of June in the Tenth year of the Reign of Our Sovereign Lady Elizabeth the Second by the Grace of God of the United Kingdom of Great Britain and Northern Ireland and of Her other Realms and Territories Queen, Head of the Commonwealth, Defender of the Faith and in the year of Our Lord One thousand nine hundred and sixty-one.

Arms of England and Scotland during our many changes of mind before final registration. The blazon reads as follows:

Per pale Sable and Argent a Chevron countercharged between in chief an Opium Poppy Flower and a Gentian Flower both slipped proper and in base a Roman Lamp Or Enflamed also proper.*

And for the Crest:

On a Wreath of the Colours an Owl proper supporting with the dexter claw a Gavel upright Or entwined with a Serpent also proper. On the dexter side a Unicorn Or armed and crined and unguled argent and on the sinister side a Lynx proper spotted Azure

---

* *The gentian.* Roger Bevan, a famous botanist and a member of our College, told us we had chosen the wrong gentian and that the one depicted on our coat of arms was different from the one used medicinally. We apologised and said if we never made a worse mistake than that we wouldn't do too badly!

Gules Vert Or and Argent and Ducally gorged and chained of the last. Motto *Cum Scientia Caritas.*†

The official blazon (Plate 21) may seem remote from the heading on notepaper and papers with which we have become so familiar since 1961 and it is interesting to recall the considerations upon which it was based. The pains of disagreement are long forgotten.

The pendant incorporating the full coat of arms was made for the College by Garrards and balances the chain superbly (Plate 22).

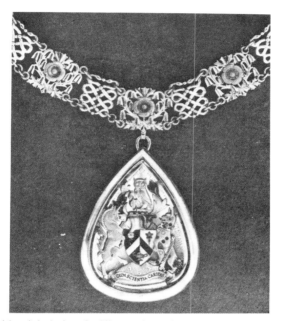

Plate 22 Presidential chain of office and pendant

A subsequent accession was a miniature badge of the same design and worn on a short ribbon of black and silver. This was easily carried in pocket or handbag and worn at distant and perhaps less formal occasions when the full badge and chain could be a burdensome responsibility.

---

† *The Crest.* Much of heraldry is based on puns. Richmond Herald was very keen that we should have an owl for our crest. We told him that we did not consider ourselves to be very clever or wise. He replied that his idea was not connected with wisdom but had to do with night calls!

The Mace

The gift of the very fine mace of silver and ebony was made by the Scottish members of College at the close of my own presidency. I remember the special pleasure of discussing with A. Donaldson in Edinburgh. He

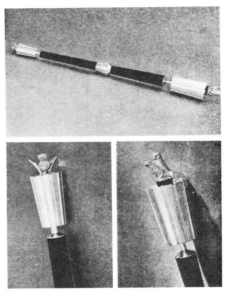

Plate 23   The College Mace

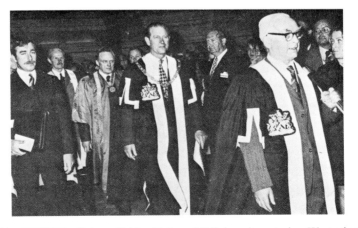

Plate 24   HRH The Prince Philip, Duke of Edinburgh, entering Westminster Hall preceded by Professor Richard Scott (Chairman of Scottish Council) bearing the College Mace

designed it with the significance of the Royal College of General Practitioners in mind. A mace is significant of the whole body on occasions where this is indicated, and is carried by the senior member of Scottish Council present at Council or Annual meetings.

The College Chaplain's Blessing of our Mace

The blessing prayer was:

> O God, who has given to men the skills of healing, and the gift of compassion, bless, we pray Thee, this Mace – a symbol of the office and work of the Royal College of General Practitioners, and grant to those who bear office in it, wisdom and right judgement. For Christ's Sake. Amen.

Academic Robes

For the President, a black union silk gown, the back being gathered on to a yoke which has no collar; the sleeves are bellshaped. The facings of the gown are trimmed in plain white ribbed silk and also around the yoke. The sleeves are trimmed at the bottom with an edging of white silk.

For members, a black gown made from a lightweight rayon fibre. The gown is fully gathered on to the yoke which has no collar. The sleeves are also gathered into the yoke. The glove sleeves are of Tudor origin and reach to within 4 inches of the hem of the gown. The ends are closed and there is an inverted 'T' shape opening at elbow level to release the arms. The facing around the yoke, opening of sleeves and slit at the sideseams are trimmed with white moiré silk.

For fellows, the gown is the same as the member's gown, but has the addition of a silk, gold and silver wire embroidered crest of the College coat of arms sewn at chest level on the right-hand side.

THE COLLEGE GRACE

The Rt. Rev. George E. Reindorp, Lord Bishop of Guildford: Salisbury

When Dame Annis Gillie became the first woman president of the College and I was the first Chaplain, she became aware that on those occasions when Grace was said before a public dinner, the form varied considerably.

It seemed to her right that the College should have a Grace of its own.

221

She asked me to compose one. This was a very tempting invitation as, from personal and sometimes painful experience, I know that Grace before an official dinner can vary from the concise and appropriate to the long-winded and inappropriate sermonette.

My naval experience reminded me of how, in various ships when they carried no parson, the Captain was wont to look round the table and say 'What, no parson – thank God!'

It was important to remember that not a few members of the College might well be of other denominations than Christian, yet all would wish to thank God for their meat in due season.

I resisted the temptation which would certainly have attracted me at a later date, when fifteen children were standing round my table with their parents and were invited to sing Grace. 'No', said a four-and-a-half-year-old twin, '*I* will say Grace.' We duly bowed our heads in a reverent Anglican manner. There was a pause. A small, clear voice said: 'God bless this bunch as they munch their lunch'. This Grace has reached a fairly wide public ever since and achieved singular fame by being related at a rather formal Royal occasion.

After suitable thought I offered to Dame Annis:

> God be praised for food and friends.
> Inspire our skills.
> Kindle our compassion.   Amen.

She approved it.

I had the Grace inscribed on a metal plate, duly mounted on wood, and presented it to the College to aid the Presidents or Chaplains who might come after me.

I am glad to note that it is becoming known throughout the various faculties of the College.

XX
RELATIONS WITH OTHER BODIES

PART I: THE MINISTRY OF HEALTH AND LATER THE DEPARTMENT OF HEALTH AND SOCIAL SECURITY

Sir George Godber

Sir Wilson Jameson, a former Chief Medical Officer and at the time Master of the Worshipful Society of Apothecaries, a long-time friend of the first President, William Pickles, played an important part in the preparatory work for the College. At that stage, however, there was little direct contact with the Ministry of Health, predecessor of the Department of Health and Social Security. There were informal contacts on a personal basis with senior medical staff who happened to be on close and friendly terms with the first officers of the College. The main formal contacts of the Department were with the General Medical Services Committee of the British Medical Association on medico-political matters from which the College studiously remained at a distance.

The first formal encounter for the College with the Ministry of Health in 1954 brought John Hunt, Donald Crombie, Robin Pinsent and Ian Watson to represent the importance of research in the future of general practice. They wanted to see a general practice member of the Medical Research Council; but in that they are still disappointed, even though Council set up a committee on research in general practice under the chairmanship of Sir Wilson Jameson.

One of the earliest examples of collaboration with the Ministry came in research when F. Scott of Ashford sought help over his survey of the

223

prevalence of macrocytic anaemia, in 1955. During the 1960s research projects of both faculties and individual members of the College increasingly received help and financial support from the Department, which greatly strengthened its involvement in research. In 1966 it was agreed to meet the greater part of the running costs of the Research and Records Unit which had been set up in Birmingham with an initial grant from the Nuffield Provincial Hospitals Trust. The weekly returns from this unit soon began to make an essential contribution to the Department's monitoring of infectious disease, especially influenza. Later the possibility of using the resources of the unit to help identify adverse reactions to prescribed drugs was to be explored with the Department's Medicines Division.

DEPARTMENT STAFF

Some of the new recruits to the Department's staff were active in the College. T. E. A. Carr was Provost of a faculty and served for two years on the Council; T. S. Eimerl had been the designer of the 'E' Book for maintaining practice disease indexes; Talbot Rogers, a founder member of the Council, was from 1963 Adviser on General Practice, part-time for five years. Since 1964 members of the Department's staff have attended main committees of the Council as invited observers.

COLLEGE MEMBERSHIP OF COMMITTEES

Within three years of its foundation the College began to be invited to give evidence to Departmental Committees, such as the Willink Committee on medical manpower and the Cranbrook Committee on the maternity services. It was natural therefore that when the Standing Medical Advisory Committee set up a subcommittee to examine the field of work of the general practitioner, Dr (now Dame) Annis Gillie, the current Chairman of the College Council and a member of the Committee, was made Chairman of the new subcommittee. Four other members of the College Council were members of this subcommittee. With increasing personal contacts between officers of the College and Departmental staff and the growing concern for improvement in general practice it became customary to seek the College's views on any matters not solely the province of the General Medical Services Committee.

The College's primary concern with education for practice made it an essential source of advice to the Ministry, as the movement for better postgraduate training spread. The recommendations of Lord Cohen's British Medical Association Committee had not been implemented, but some regions began to look for opportunities to establish joint training posts in hospitals and general practice. The Conference on Postgraduate Medical Education at Christ Church, Oxford, organized by the Nuffield Provincial Hospitals Trust in 1961, was a turning point. The Presidents of the College and the, then, three Royal Colleges, the Secretary and Chief Medical Officer of the Ministry, and the President of the General Medical Council, were among those who met under Sir George Pickering's chairmanship. Publication of the conclusions by the Chairman was at once followed by a promise of financial support from the Nuffield Provincial Hospitals Trust and met such a response from the profession as no other initiative linked with the National Health Service has evoked.

Within two years not only had many postgraduate centres been established at district hospitals but National Health Service funds had been committed to their provision and support. Although the original intention had been linked at least as much with training in the hospital specialties, the greatest response came from general practice and especially from College members. From then on, increasingly close collaboration, without encroaching on the independence of the College, became essential. Although legitimate General Medical Services Committee interests were jealously safeguarded, there was no doubt whence the main influence on Departmental thinking about preparation for general practice came. For instance the Graves Medical Audiovisual Library grew up within the College with a modest Departmental grant.

MORE RESEARCH

The College's contribution to research has been of the utmost importance. Without it no such large-scale studies as that on the safety of oral contraception could have been undertaken. The network of recording practices, established by the Birmingham Research Unit, provided the necessary base for the first and second National Morbidity Surveys. The latter, in 1970/71, organized jointly by the College, Department of Health and Social Security and Office of Population Censuses and Surveys, is likely to be used for the third survey being planned. The development of health education in general practice has also been helped by representation of the College on the Health Education Council.

COLLEGE REPORTS AND THE CHARTER

Negotiations for the General Practice Charter in the 1960s were a General Medical Services Committee affair, but they were much influenced by such factual College publications as the first report (1965) on *Present State and Future Needs of General Practice*. The College had been represented in the earlier Fraser Working Party which had done some of the groundwork for the later discussions on the Charter. The College *Journal* and many special reports were a principal source of new initiatives in general practice. At the same time it has become increasingly common for Departmental staff to take part in College symposia.

The long struggle for mandatory vocational training for general practice was largely initiated by the College but welcomed by the Department. The College was rightly represented on the Council for Post-graduate Medical Education from the outset. Development of the necessary organization to sustain vocational training, training of general-practitioner trainers, and the setting-up of a network of training schemes could not have begun until the Charter provided a suitable financial basis. It was also necessary to have the painstaking appraisal of the effectiveness of training undertaken with Department of Health and Social Security support by Professor Patrick Byrne's Unit at Manchester. The common interest of the College and Department was also essential in solving the problems which arose during the eight years of preparation through the framing of the Act, the establishment of the Joint Committee for Postgraduate Training in General Practice and the framing and implementation of the detailed regulations. It may well be that the informality of relations was a condition of success.

A JOINT WORKING PARTY

It was on the initiative of the College that a Joint Working Party was set up by the Department of Health and Social Security, General Medical Services Committee and the College in 1972 to 'consider National Health Service general practice as it is developing now and as it should be assisted to develop in the future'. That followed the first two Cogwheel Reports on medical work in hospitals and it was hoped that other reports would follow the first which was published in 1974. Unhappily the worsening relation-ships in the National Health Service impeded this; but good personal contacts remained, and through these much has been achieved despite the limited formal consultation. There may indeed be better methods.

THE FUTURE

Now, after its first 25 years, the position of the Royal College of General Practitioners as standard-setter in general medical practice is as firmly established as are those of the older Royal Colleges in their special fields. Department of Health and Social Security co-operation is therefore assured in the interests of the National Health Service and is all the more effective because money is never a factor in securing it. The independence of the College position is absolutely essential to its strength, but that in no way precludes a sensible and co-operative relationship with the main government agency concerned.

PART II: THE BRITISH MEDICAL ASSOCIATION AND ITS GENERAL MEDICAL SERVICES COMMITTEE

Ekke V. Kuenssberg

During the College's early days the BMA, mainly through its Journal, was an essential help in focusing the minds of those engaged in shaping its future. Once the College was launched and it became clear to all those interested that it was not going to interfere in the affairs of the BMA or the GMSC but would keep itself to education and research, we had much continuing support – the *BMJ* carrying long reports of College symposia, its Annual General Meetings and the first Mackenzie Lectures. This was indeed personified by the Foundation Council's membership of four outstanding BMA activists – Fraser Rose, Ian Grant, Annis Gillie and Talbot Rogers – the first three of whom later became Presidents of the College. Fraser Rose's influence in bringing much of the BMA statutes to the College is discussed elsewhere. Ian Grant's death deprived the College of a powerful medico-political figure, whose period of Chairman of Council of the BMA fell in a time of very active College growth, which might well have led to misunderstanding with less far-sighted medical statesmen. The research work and organizational studies carried out by the College began to be of some help during such BMA/GMSC occasions as the Fraser Committee 1962 and the Charter negotiations in 1964–66.

It was inevitable that we should have a deep crisis. In 1965, during the Swansea BMA meeting, a reporter working for the *Daily Express* obtained a prepublication copy (still under embargo) of the first attempt by the College at surveying general practice. An unfortunate interview, unrehearsed and unprepared, about selected excerpts from the first 'Present State and Future Needs of General Practice' gave a bored press three-inch headlines and the BMA correspondence column much venom. The leading article in the *BMJ* (July 24 1965) attempted, in sorrow rather than in anger, to refute what had been stirred up, and was under the circumstances a most thoughtful analysis. What appeared to be so unacceptable then, is today recognized as fact. But then the years 1964–66 were medico-politically hightide years, when emotive behaviour was all too readily accepted. A joint letter in August of 1965 attempted, successfully, to lower the fever heat between the organizations. It was signed by Annis Gillie as President of the College of General Practitioners, Harry Levitt as Chairman of Council, J. R. Nicholson Lailey, Chairman of the BMA Council and J. C. Cameron, Chairman of the GMSC. The last two paragraphs read:

> On behalf of the Council of the College we wish to make it clear that the College has no wish or intention to exceed its proper academic activity of investigating and improving standards of general practice or to take part in medicopolitical affairs. Moreover, we both wish to strengthen our relationship by improving the arrangements for liaison which already exist between our two bodies.
>
> The College and the BMA have a common aim. It is to do everything possible to improve standards and conditions in general practice. We hope that this joint letter will serve as an indication of our firm resolve.

The next crisis was not long in coming, although the GMSC and the College kept meeting in a Liaison Committee three or four times a year. The BMA and the GMSC, as well as the *British Medical Journal*, did not see the need for the development of an examination. While the College membership itself was split on this, the gentle, or at times raucous, advice from local medical committees and their Conference was not too flattering.

Yet it was not long before the goodwill of these organizations was restored, particularly after the Royal Commission on Medical Education (Todd) reported, accepting and recommending the line of evidence submitted by the College. Since then there have been a number of occasions of most constructive co-operation when the two bodies – the GMSC and the College – have produced outstanding results in cross-fertilization and support. In one particular area the College's contribution to the BMA/GMSC problems has been widely appreciated. The entry into the European Economic Community presented the UK general practitioners with many possible problems and solutions and, through the College's accepted educational evidence and expertise, it was possible to give the many UK proposals firm factual backing, in particular through the organization of the Union Européenne des Médecins Omnipraticiens (UEMO), being the GP national representatives, hopefully advising the Council of Europe and its Brussels organization.

The development of the Postgraduate Council, with its General Practice Advisory Committee with equal membership from both organizations, the Godber Committee enquiring and eventually reporting in 1973 on some of the outstanding problems of general medical services, the Joint GMSC/RCGP committee on Medical Records, are other examples of good co-operation; and, finally, since 1976 the Joint Committee on Post-graduate Training for General Practice has in its bipartite membership led to the setting up of mandatory vocational training for principals in the National Heath Service.

XXI
THE COLLEGE OVERSEAS

OVERSEAS REGIONAL FACULTIES

John H. Hunt, John A. R. Lawson and Ian R. McWhinney

From the College's earliest days, the Steering Committee had planned to encourage the development of overseas regional faculties in Australia, New Zealand and later on in South Africa, with their corresponding Overseas Regional Councils. As with the home faculties the Officers and Members of Faculty Boards are printed in the *Annual Reports*. The Foundation Council agreed that at least ten members of the College would be needed to form an overseas faculty and that the College Council should decide the area to be covered by each.

By the time the College was a year old, two overseas faculties were in being. By the end of its fifth year there were ten. The remarkable early achievements of these overseas faculties, encouraging general practice in their areas, are well described in a report from each published at the end of each *Annual Report* of the College.

OVERSEAS MEMBERS AND ASSOCIATES WHO DID NOT BELONG TO A FACULTY

Many members and associates joined the College from countries where there were no overseas faculties or before they had been formed, as from South Africa and Kenya. The number of these other countries they came from astonished us. One of the most unusual was Victor Smolnikoff from Moscow. He had worked in a successful general practice in Shanghai when

231

he was invited to return to Russia as a senior anaesthetist, because he had been able to master the use of the Boyle's anaesthetic machine. So he moved to Moscow with all his family and belongings which included a grand piano! He wrote to us to say he wanted to join the College and enclosed a money order for £50 in return for which he said he hoped we would make him a life member, which we did. John Hunt visited him in his flat in Moscow five years later.

Other overseas members and associates not then attached to a faculty were working in Malta (1), Austria (1), India (11), Ceylon (8), Burma (3), Malaya (16), Assam (1), Borneo (1), Hong Kong (1), Iraq (1), Canada (13), USA (3), British West Indies (2), The Falkland Islands (1), Union of South Africa (6), Kenya (14), Southern Rhodesia (9), South West Africa (1), Tanganyika (1), French Equatorial Africa (1), Belgian Congo (1), British Cameroons (2), Gold Coast (1), Nigeria (3), and Sierre Leone (1). This was a good example of widespread interest in the College.

In 1968 Ian R. McWhinney went to London, Ontario, as Professor of Family Medicine, where he still does active work for our College.

OVERSEAS COUNCILS

THE AUSTRALIAN COUNCIL

W. A. Conolly and H. Stuart Patterson
In the summer of 1952 W. A. Conolly met John Hunt in London and learned of the proposal to form a College of General Practitioners. He wrote a letter to the *British Medical Journal* in support and, when the College of General Practitioners was founded on November 19 1952, many family doctors in Australia became foundation members. Interest soon grew, particularly in New South Wales and Queensland. On October 30 1953 the New South Wales faculty was established, only six months after the first faculty in Britain and seven months before any of the four London faculties. The following year, on August 27 1954, under the guiding hand of Stuart Patterson, the first meeting of the Queensland faculty was held.

Initially there was some opposition to the formation of an independent body representing general practitioners in Australia, and there was also opposition from the Federal Council of the British Medical Association there. It was feared that this branch of the new college was to be medico-political and might embarrass the Australian Medical Association. Dr Stuart Patterson (at that time President of the Queensland branch of the BMA) was asked by the Federal Council for a report on the aims of the College. When, as a result of this report, it was realized that the interests of the College were purely academic, the opposition of the Federal Council disappeared.

It is also of some historical interest to record that from the earliest years some of the keener minds amongst general practitioners in Australia recognized the need for a higher qualification in general practice. As far back as 1955 the minutes of the Queensland faculty state that such a recommendation was sent to the Postgraduate Medical Education Committee of the University of Queensland. Subsequently, in 1956, the Australian Council recommended to College Council that consideration be given to an examination for membership which was essential to promote equality with the other colleges and to give the new College pride in itself.

At the time of the Australasian Congress of the British Medical Association held in Sydney in August 1955, the New South Wales faculty held a special general meeting attended by members from all parts of the continent to discuss the future of the College in Australia. Also attending was A. Talbot Rogers, who was representing the British College of General Practitioners as well as the British Medical Association. The meeting resolved that the New South Wales faculty board should take the necessary steps to constitute an Australian Council of the College and that arrangements be left in the hands of its chairman, W. A. Conolly. Dr Talbot Rogers warmly supported this decision.

On September 4 1955, a meeting took place at the United Service Club, Brisbane. It was attended by W. A. Conolly and H. M. Saxby (representing the New South Wales faculty) and Stuart Patterson, B. N. Adsett and W. J. Hamilton (representing the Queensland faculty). It was decided to form an Australian Council of the College. This was approved at the Annual General Meeting of the College in London on November 19 1955. The following were elected to office: Chairman: W. A. Conolly (New South Wales), Vice-chairman: H. S. Patterson (Queensland), Honorary Secretary: H. M. Saxby (New South Wales), Members: B. N. Adsett (Queensland), W. J. Hamilton (Queensland), C. W. Anderson (Western Australia), D. M. Clement (Western Australia), H. E. H. Ferguson (Western Australia) and C. Warburton (New South Wales).

In its early days the Australian Council recorded its debt of gratitude to College Council for its grant of £200 and the provision of a typewriter and duplicating machine. It was also very appreciative of the assistance and guidance it had received from College Council and in particular from John Hunt and Commander A. E. P. Doran.

Although, at the time it was decided to establish an Australian Council, the only faculties in Australia were those in New South Wales and Queensland, there was considerable interest in the other states, particularly

Western Australia. The *Western Australia faculty* was established on January 18 1956.

On August 15 1956, at a meeting of the Council of the Australian College held at Lismore, New South Wales, a policy for the future development of the College in Australia was formulated and arrangements were made for Dr Saxby to visit the states in which faculties had not yet been established. Thanks largely to the assistance of the state branches of the BMA, successful meetings were held in Melbourne, Hobart and Adelaide. The *Victoria faculty* was formed at a meeting held in Melbourne on November 1 1956, and Roy Bartram, David Zacharin and G.D. McDonald were elected members of the Australian Council. In Tasmania a General Practitioner Group had been formed on November 22 1953, and on November 20 1955 the Group recommended that its members join the College of General Practitioners. The *Tasmania faculty* was formally inaugurated at a meeting in Hobart on May 5 1957, with Shad Saxby (honorary secretary of the Australian Council) and others in attendance. Trevor James was elected Provost and Chairman, R.J.D. Turnbull the Honorary Secretary, and Athol Corney the Honorary Treasurer. These members were also elected to the Australian Council.

The only Australian state which had not yet established a faculty was South Australia, but interest there was growing so Dr Saxby paid a visit to Adelaide, interviewed several leading general practitioners and, finally, on February 8 1958, the *South Australia faculty* was formed. Forthwith C.C. Jungfer, D.K. Kumnick and L.R. Mallen were elected members of the Australian Council.

During 1957 the bye-laws for the Australian Council were submitted to and approved by College Council. Chairmen were appointed to the Committees of Council as follows: Undergraduate Education (T.E.Y Holcombe), Postgraduate Education (C. Warburton) and Research (J.G. Radford). Meantime, the New South Wales, Queensland and Western Australian faculties had initiated publication of the first official journal of the College in Australia – *Annals of General Practice* – with Carl Gunther as editor and chairman of the Editorial Committee.

In Australia the College was quickly coming to be recognized. In 1957 the Australian Government invited the Australian Council of the College to nominate a member of the College for appointment to the National Health and Medical Research Council. J.G. Radford was put forward and duly appointed to this important body. In the same year the Minister for Health of the Australian Government, the Hon Donald Cameron, OBE, suggested that the Australian Council of the College should set up a permanent Committee in Preventive Medicine in addition to its other standing committees. He believed this committee could perform a most useful function as a link between the Commonwealth Department of Health and general practitioners. The first chairman of this Preventive Medicine Committee, set up in 1958, was C. C. Jungfer and the committee has remained in existence ever since. It has proved a great success. Meantime C. Jungfer, who had visited Canada, the United States and the United Kingdom obtaining information about surveys of general practice in those countries, carried out a survey himself of Australian general practice, which was largely financed by the Australian Government and made with the co-operation of the Federal Council of the British Medical Association[1]. His report was to prove most helpful in the future activities of the College in Australia.

During its first two years the Australian Council was largely financed by the New South Wales faculty, sharing its secretariat and headquarters, which were in rooms of a College member, C. W. F. Laidlaw.

Consideration had been given to the founding of an independent Australian College of General Practitioners as far back as 1953. Now, partly for geographical reasons and partly because of the differences between general practice in Australia and the United Kingdom, it was felt the time was approaching to bring this to fruition. To be certain that Australian members of the College were in favour of the formation of an Australian College of General Practitioners, a questionnaire was sent to them. With very few exceptions, members said there should be an Australian College which should function from July 1 1958.

On February 4 1958, with the consent and blessing of the British College, the *Australian College of General Practitioners* was incorporated and the final meeting of the Australian Council of the British College, held in Hobart on March 6 1958, resolved that it would be dissolved as from June 30 1958 and that the necessary actions would be taken to allow the Australian College of General Practitioners to function from July 1 1958.

Deep appreciation of the generosity of the Council of the British College of General Practitioners was recorded thus:

Not only was valuable equipment transferred to this [the Australian] College but also considerable funds became the property of the Council [of the Australian College] and its faculties. But, more than this material generosity, the spirit of goodwill and sympathetic interest were at all times most impressive. This College commenced its independent life with the knowledge that it could always rely on the guidance and goodwill of a wise and generous parent. May we always be worthy of that parentage and may the achievement of the passing years strengthen the filial bonds.

235

Membership of the British College in Australia on June 30 1958, was 761.

Chairman of Australian Council

W. A. Conolly 1955

THE NEW ZEALAND COUNCIL

C. L. E. L. Sheppard

In New Zealand, several general practitioners joined the British College soon after its foundation, and on November 12 1953 A. B. Jameson and T. D. C. Childs formed the first faculty of the College in New Zealand, the *Auckland faculty*, with 30 members and three associates.

In 1954, C. L. E. L. Sheppard of Christchurch was in Glasgow as a New Zealand delegate to the British Medical Association and met John Hunt, Ian Grant, Fraser Rose and other foundation members of the College. He became an associate of the College and was convinced of the important place the College was to take in the future of medical practice in New Zealand. Early in 1955 a meeting was arranged for general practitioners in Christchurch and it was decided to set up the *Canterbury faculty.*

Later, in 1955, interest in the College led to the establishment of the *Otago faculty* in Dunedin. On December 14 1955, A. B. Jameson, Chairman of the Auckland faculty, invited the Chairmen and Secretaries of the Canterbury and Otago faculties to meet him and Dr Childs, the Secretary of the Auckland faculty, in Wellington to establish an interim New Zealand Council of the College of General Practitioners. All agreed to establish the Interim Council and provisional bye-laws were drawn up.

In 1956 the *Wellington faculty* was established.

New Zealand Council met on June 15 1956, in Wellington, and plans for the future of the College in New Zealand were discussed. It was decided to hold the first meeting of New Zealand members and associates in Wellington on February 19 1957. At this meeting the Interim New Zealand Council was dissolved and C. L. E. L. Sheppard was elected Chairman and L. H. Cordery Honorary Secretary of the *New Zealand Council of the British College of General Practitioners.*

It was decided that the headquarters of the Council would be sited for a period of two years in turn in the faculties – until May 1959 in Canterbury, until 1961 in Auckland, until 1963 in Otago and then until 1965 in Wellington. At this stage, September 30 1957, there were 103 members and 22 associates, a total of 125 registered in New Zealand. A uniform system of payment of fees was introduced and the transmission of funds to the College Council in London was adopted. The New Zealand Council agreed to the College Council's policy of the distribution of entrance fees and annual subscriptions between the College Council and the New Zealand Council and faculties. Gratitude was expressed to the College Council for its grant of £100 to help in establishing the secretariat in New Zealand.

The New Zealand Council was to coordinate the work between the four faculties and the British Council and keep it informed of the special needs of New Zealand.

Suggestions for criteria for membership and associateship were made and sent to the College Council for consideration and approval and a scheme for general-practitioner training for final year medical students was being implemented in the faculties.

The New Zealand Council recorded its appreciation for the help it had received from the College Council and especially from John Hunt, Sylvia Chapman and Commander A. E. P. Doran. It was also grateful for the co-operation of the New Zealand faculties and the New Zealand branch of the British Medical Association.

Progress in the College was steady and activities led to the first College congress in Christchurch on February 10–13 1959, held in conjunction with the British Medical Association biennial conference. The guests were I. .D. Grant, President of the College, H. M. Saxby, Honorary Secretary of the Australian College Council, and H. C. Fox representing the American Academy of General Practice. The congress was a success and attracted a large attendance of members and non-members.

Following a visit to all New Zealand faculties, Ian Grant went to Sydney, Australia, where he formally established The Australian College of General Practitioners by handing over control from the College in Britain. Following that conference, in recognition of their outstanding services to the College, Honorary Fellowship of the British College was granted to A. B. Jameson (Auckland) and L. H. Cordery (Canterbury).

In September 1959 the headquarters of the New Zealand College Council transferred to the Auckland faculty, with T. D. S. Childs as Chairman and D. C. Campbell as Honorary Secretary.

Council and faculties made steady progress and their planning led to a College congress in Auckland in February 1961. Guests were J. H. Hunt representing the British Council, E. C. McCoy representing the Canadian Academy of General Practitioners and C. L. Howe representing the Australian College of General Practitioners.

In September 1961 the headquarters of the New Zealand College Council transferred to the Otago faculty, with H. E. M. Williams as Chairman and A. Borrie as Honorary Secretary.

Activities continued in establishing the position of the College and led to the congress in Dunedin on February 10–11 1963. The guests were George Swift representing the College Council, Stuart Patterson representing the Australian College and Dr Margaret Donnell representing the Canadian Academy of General Practitioners.

In September 1963 the headquarters of the Council transferred to the Wellington faculty, with P. D. Delany as Chairman and R. P. Tuckey as Honorary Secretary.

Council work continued and progress was made in the examination for entry and on undergraduate education.

Fellowship of the College in New Zealand by election for outstanding service to the College and medicine was introduced in June 1964.

On September 18 1965 the headquarters were transferred to the Canterbury faculty; T. K. Williams was Chairman and W. H. Brockett, Honorary Secretary.

In November 1965 there was an approach by P. D. Delany to the New Zealand Council to gain approval for the formation of an independent New Zealand College. There was discussion by the faculties. Votes were equally divided in the Council meeting, but T. K. Williams, as Chairman, gave his casting vote for the *status quo*.

In February 1967 a conference was held in Christchurch. T. S. Eimerl was a visitor from the United Kingdom College.

In September 1967 the headquarters of the College was transferred to the Auckland faculty; Chairman, W. N. Clay and Honorary Secretary, J. G. Richards. The Medical Education Committee had made progress in the criteria for membership and the examination system. Also a request was made and granted by the Medical Council of New Zealand to recognize the registration of the FRCGP and MRCGP diploma.

A congress was held in Auckland on February 9–14 1969. In July 1969 the headquarters of the College transferrred to the Otago faculty; R. D. MacDiarmid was chairman and B. B. Grimmond honorary secretary. The need for general-practitioner registrarship was recognized by H. J. H. Hiddleston, Director-General of the Health Department of New Zealand, and a pilot scheme was introduced by Eric Elder in Southland.

In September 1971, a suggestion was made that the New Zealand College of General Practitioners be launched at a conference in 1974, and C. L. E. L. Sheppard was appointed Conference Committee Chairman. In March 1972 Council decided on a postal referendum of members of the College in New Zealand on the formation of a possible New Zealand College. The vote produced over two thirds majority in favour of the move.

In July 1972 the number of doctors who joined the British College was now 37 fellows, 355 members and 96 associates – a total of 488. During 1972 the Otago faculty changed its name to the Otago–Southland Faculty and in 1973 the Waikato faculty was formed. B. H. Young was chairman.

In May 1973 the headquarters of the College transferred to the Canterbury faculty; J. P. Musgrove was chairman and R. A. Cartwright honorary secretary.

The establishment of the New Zealand College of General Practitioners was effected at a Foundation Dinner held in Christchurch on January 24 1974. His Royal Highness The Prince Philip, Duke of Edinburgh, Patron of the College, and P. S. Byrne, President, attended and formally handed over control of the New Zealand Council and faculties to the New Zealand College. P. D. Delany, the first President of the New Zealand College, accepted on behalf of the College.

The inaugural conference of the new College was held in Christchurch from February 6–13 1974. The guests present were Professor P. S. Byrne, J. Radford (President of the Royal Australian College of General Practitioners), Wong Heck Sing (President of the College of General Practitioners Singapore), P. Mehta (President of the Association of General Practitioners of Fiji), D. I. Rice (Executive Director of the Academy of Family Physicians of Canada), M. Cooling (Chairman of Council, the Royal Australian College of General Practitioners) and D. Game (President-Elect of the Royal Australian College).

The conference was judged an enjoyable and successful function and attracted a large attendance.

The New Zealand College was launched with a wealth of kindness and good wishes by our former partners in the College in Britain and by the representatives from Australia, Canada, Singapore and Fiji.

Chairmen of New Zealand Council

C. L. E. L. Sheppard	1957	T. K. Williams	1966
T. D. C. Childs	1960	W. N. Clay	1968
H. E. M. Williams	1962	R. D. MacDiarmid	1971
P. D. Delany	1964		

THE SOUTH AFRICAN COUNCIL

F. E. Hofmeyr

After a successful Medical Congress in Durban in 1957, the Congress President (Professor H. Grant-Whyte), noticed that no provision had been made for the general practitioner. With the surplus funds Professor Grant-Whyte, who had knowledge of the problems of general practice, arranged for the then President of the British College of General Practitioners (Ian

D. Grant) to visit South Africa in 1958 and lecture on the College's activities at all the major centres. The National General Practitioner's Group, under the chairmanship of George Paterson, organized the venues. The dynamic lectures of Dr Grant were well attended. It was clear that the problems of general practice in Britain had been very similar to those in South Africa where the specialist was taking control of the practice of medicine.

Great interest was aroused amongst the general practitioners at a meeting held on September 30 1958, in Pretoria, attended by I. D. Grant. It was decided that Regional Faculties of the College should be formed in South Africa, and very many South African doctors joined the College. On November 21 1958 the *Witwatersrand faculty* was founded. In June 1959 the *Cape of Good Hope faculty* was formed, followed by the *Natal* faculty on March 8 1960, and later the *Orange Free State*, *Cape Eastern* and *Northern Transvaal* faculties. The strict requirements for membership, including having been in active general practice for the previous five years and an undertaking to do at least 25 hours postgraduate study every two years and to practise medicine of a high ethical standard as judged by one's colleagues, appealed to many doctors.

The need to coordinate, supervise and stimulate the activities led to the formation of an *Interim South African Council* on October 19 1960, at a meeting in Vereeniging with F. E. Hofmeyr as chairman and A. G. Paterson as secretary. Also at that historic meeting were D. H. Pirie, S. J. Lachman, E. S. W. Deale, A. Broomberg, J. van der Riet, P. D. Beck and A. P. Albert and, as observers, Professor H. Grant-Whyte, Professor H. A. Shapiro and Drs N. Levy and C. L. Grobler.

In Pretoria great success was achieved through the farsightedness of Professor H. W. Snyman who, with H. P. Botha, established a Department of General Practice in the Medical School. Dr Botha became its first professor and the department awarded the degree of MMed(Prax), approved by the South African Medical and Dental Council. Today this is a department with international recognition.

The membership of the British College in South Africa grew. Its activities increased and it became recognized and respected throughout the country. The help given by Ian Grant until his death in 1961, and also that of John Hunt, John Fry, the Canadian Donald Rice, and E. V. Kuenssberg must be recorded. Membership reached several hundreds. It was not surprising that at a full South African Council meeting in October 1967 it was formally proposed that an independent South African College should be formed. This decision was communicated to the Council of the Royal College and John Hunt kindly proposed at the Annual General Meeting on November 18 1967, that 'this College welcomes the proposal that a College of General Practitioners be founded in South Africa in 1968'. At the next meeting of the full South African Council, in Cape Town on May 31 1968, the resolution to establish a South African College of General Practitioners was formally adopted. F. E. Hofmeyr (Chairman of the South African Council), N. Levy (Honorary Secretary) and W. A. Miller (a leading member of the Transvaal faculty) were appointed trustees to act for the South African College until it was duly registered. Drs Hofmeyr, Levy and Miller had recently been honoured by being elected Fellows of the now Royal College of General Practitioners in Britain; other members to be elected fellows were H. P. Botha, J. A. Smith, B. M. Fehler, G. Daynes and B. Jaffe.

The independent College of General Practitioners of South Africa was formed with its headquarters in Cape Town, and owed its strength and success in no small measure to the valuable assistance from Mrs Audrey Benjamin and Mrs Helen Harbottle, and from the office staff of the British Royal College of General Practitioners and, in particular, to Ian Grant and John Hunt.

The names of all those who played leading parts in the foundation of the South African faculties and of the South African College may be found in the British College's *Annual Reports*.

The College of General Practitioners of South Africa was successful as an independent College. Later it amalgamated with the College of Physicians, Surgeons, Obstetricians and Gynaecologists to form the College of Medicine in South Africa. This was the first College to have all the disciplines under one roof.

Chairman of South African Council

F. E. Hofmeyr 1961

Reference

1. Conolly, W. A. (1952) College of General Practice. *Br.Med. J.,* **ii,** 444

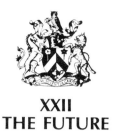

XXII
THE FUTURE

PART I: THE FUTURE OF THE COLLEGE IN HEALTH CARE IN GENERAL AND OF PRIMARY CARE

John Fry and Gordon McLachlan

The past is history. Now after more than 25 years the College looks to the future to play its part in promoting high standards of care and service.

Our roles in the future can be examined under three headings – the future of health, the future of primary care and the future of the Royal College of General Practitioners.

THE FUTURE OF HEALTH CARE IN GENERAL

The provision of good health care demands huge coordinated efforts between professional and technical workers, the public and lay workers, families and individuals, and between governments and other funding organizations.

Within the health-care system, primary care (general practice) is essential and inevitable in every national health system. It is not possible, and quite wrong, to consider general practice in isolation yet, paradoxically, it is important to grant it independent and distinct status.

General practice is a horizontal level of care, just as are self-care and specialist care. It has its own ethos and its own scientific core of knowledge that has to be researched, taught, learnt and applied, as have its methods and techniques of work, and its own systems of assessment and standards.

Its special strengths are to provide constant available, accessible, continuing, personal and family health care with attention to its physical, behavioural, social and preventive aspects.

In stating the special distinctness of general practice it is important to stress its essential unity with all the other medical, paramedical and lay groups involved in a modern health system.

Our immediate future is filled with challenge, difficulties and dilemmas. Better health has to be based on:

(1) Health promotion through education of and information for the public as well as professional health workers.

(2) Health maintenance involving individual responsibilities in taking steps to keep fit and avoid accidents and disease, as well as professional and governmental responsibilities in providing resources.

(3) Better protection against diseases and their care by medical and social progress based on research and evaluation of therapeutic methods.

(4) Prevention involving personal, family and public involvement.

There are finite limits to the amount of money, manpower and other resources that can be given to health care.

With increasing worldwide economic difficulties, financial limits on health resources are inevitable. There will be increasing need to avoid waste and unnecessary use of medical resources such as prescribing of unnecessary drugs, unnecessary investigations, unnecessary hospitalization and wasteful systems of organization and administration. Within a finite economic system there will have to be controls, rationing and priorities.

The Future Of Primary Care

As the largest section within the medical profession and as the most important portal of entry into the health-care system, general practice will have special responsibilities in playing its part in providing better health for the people in a better and sharper and more effective, efficient and economic health service.

World Scene

Better primary care has been recognized by the World Health Organization

(WHO) as the most hopeful factor for providing 'health for all' in the world by the year 2000. Affirmation of WHO policy to promote and support primary care was achieved through the Alma Ata Declaration at a WHO conference at Alma Ata in the USSR in 1978.

The problems, deficiencies and needs of primary care all over the world are receiving attention and support. The College, through its own work and experience and through its participation in the work of the World Organization of National Colleges and Academies of General Practice/Family Medicine (WONCA), will have much to contribute in the international field.

United Kingdom

Pessimists over the past 30 years have frequently forecast the demise of general practice in the United Kingdom and noted its supposed irrelevance in the modern medical scene.

Yet the first 25 years of the College's existence have watched general practice grow in strength and importance. General practice is the oldest specialty. It has existed ever since medical care began. There always has been the need for some physician to provide primary general continuing care for individuals and families. The College may be less than 40 years old now; primary care goes back to the early development of the human race.

Future trends are rooted in a fertile past. The roots of British general practice are long and firm. The tradition of the general practitioner – family doctor working on his own and providing primary and continuing care both in general and specialist fields goes back to the early nineteenth century.

Solo practice was customary until the 1950s. Until then more than four out of five British general practitioners were working on their own, usually from their own homes, often with their wives acting as unpaid receptionists, secretaries, book-keepers, dispensers or nurses. There were few partnerships or rota arrangements, and holidays meant a search for a locum, or some arrangement with a neighbouring practitioner, which sometimes led to anxieties over losing patients to local competitors.

It was with the introduction of the British National Health Service, in 1948, that major changes began to occur. By virtue of the capitation system of remuneration and financial inducements to share premises, form groups of three or more doctors and employ practice staff, competition for patients declined and better-planned organization of work became possible.

In the past 25 years the following trends in British general practice have been notable:

(1) Maintenance of the *independent contractual status* of the general practitioner.

(2) *Small group practice* (in 1980 only 15% of general practitioners worked solo and more than one-half in groups of three or more doctors). The average size of a group was between three and four, showing that there was no trend to very large groups.

(3) *Teamwork* – almost all general practices now employ secretarial, receptionist and other staff. Nurses, health visitors, midwives, social workers and some other paramedical workers are attached to general practices and there is collaboration and co-operation within the community.

(4) *Health centres* – from a handful of purpose-built health centres there are now more than 1250 housing about 25% of all general practitioners.

(5) *Work outside general practice*. About 9000 general practitioners, one third of the total, worked part-time in NHS hospital appointments as members of specialist units and others used local hospitals to care for their own patients. Many general practitioners served as industrial medical officers, as medical examiners for insurance and government organizations, in teaching and training and in other capacities. General practice is now a part-time occupation for most practitioners.

(6) *As a specialty*, general practice will require a mandatory three-year period of *vocational training* from now on. An annual output of 1200–1500 new general practitioners means that at any time there will be up to 4500 young doctors in training.

(7) There are *departments of general practice* at most British medical schools, and *continuing education* is an everyday component of one's work – from clinical experience, reading and study, from small group meetings and from formal educational sessions at district postgraduate medical centres.

Within this history of progress and success there are some current problems that will continue into the future and pose challenges.

(1) *Standards and quality of care and service.*
    Having established a recognizable field within medicine with its own educational base, general practice and its College must next be concerned with ensuring and maintaining good standards of service and care for the public. It would be best for all if such tasks

were undertaken by the profession itself rather than imposed upon it from outside. Within the British medical system there are statutory bodies such as the General Medical Council, Family Practitioner Committees and Courts that ensure professional modes of behaviour and service; but these work broadly and act only when complaints are brought to them.

It is up to the medical profession, general practice and the College to create more specific and detailed ways of assessing standards within general practice by non-threatening and non-punitive means, and to encourage and promote better care and service. In addition to audits, checks, assessments and other measurements of quality and standards, there is need for incentives and rewards to encourage better care and service. The most effective ways of achieving these are to incorporate such incentives and rewards into the system of remuneration, where proven and exceptional methods of care and service earn extra fees.

(2) *Specialization within general practice* is a matter that may require resolution. General practice must continue to remain primarily a generalist horizontal service providing general care for all problems and all people, within the practitioner's capabilities. There is no reason why practitioners, within it, should not develop their own special skills and interests. These should be complementary to their normal service to their patients.

(3) *Relations with other specialists* must continue at their present good levels and be developed further. General practice is the only truly general clinical specialty. General practitioners have the traditional role of primary physicians. They will receive, assess and manage their patients at the first professional level. Their good relations with other specialists must be based on a system of referral to and referral back to the general practitioner, when the specialist has completed his work.

(4) *The public, patients, families and individuals* are an essential part of the health care system. *Self-care* is the true first level of care and the great majority of minor maladies and chronic disorders are cared for by individuals and families themselves without frequent recourse to general practitioners or specialists. Good care and service depends on good relations between the public and general practice. It is the duty of all doctors to teach and inform their patients and to motivate them to collaborate and to participate in their own care. In the future there will be need to create even better

and more formal relationships between general practices and their communities through patient groups and other means.

The first 25 years of the Royal College of General Practitioners laid the pattern for its future work and development. It has a sound central organization. Yet the full flowering of the College's potential depends on the involvement and participation of individual members at local faculty and subfaculty levels.

The College must be outward looking and, through its members, be involved in national and local medical and extramedical affairs that can enhance the status of general practice and its quality of care and service.

The College has created admirable and admired examples of professional leadership in international as well as in national fields. As a high priority it must continue to develop intra- and interprofessional relations with:

(1) other Colleges and professional organizations at home and abroad;
(2) other sister professions;
(3) other academic and industrial organizations;
(4) the public;
(5) the Government.

In its more specific professional work it has long established functional activities within its organization. The Education Committee, for example, with its long record of achievements, can now leave undergraduate and vocational education to the universities and to regional and local vocational-training programmes, supported by an examination for membership of the College. A high priority must be continuing education as a means of improving standards of care and service.

The Practice Organization Committee and its successor will continue to be involved in collecting data on what goes on in general practice and in providing advice and information for those who seek it.

Research in, and into, general practice has much to offer in the future. In spite of the work of individuals there is still much that is unknown and undiscovered in general practice. More clinical research to increase our knowledge of the nature, course, outcome and response to treatment of common diseases is urgently necessary.

Facts and data on care, management and outcome of behavioural, psychological and social problems are deficient. Information on efficiency, efficacy and economics of our practice organization is almost non-existent.

The core of knowledge in general practice has to be:

(1) researched, analysed and discussed,
(2) taught and learnt,

(3) applied and practised,

(4) continually reassessed and checked.

Some of these points are discussed by Sir George Godber in the second part of this chapter.

PART II: THE FUTURE OF THE ROYAL COLLEGE OF GENERAL PRACTITIONERS

Sir George Godber

General medical practice occupies a more secure position in the United Kingdom than in many other countries. Its form has changed substantially during the lifetime of the College and the changes have been largely influenced by the work of the College. Without its becoming involved in medicopolitical or financial negotiations the respect accorded to the College has ensured that its views substantially determine the principles upon which such innovations as compulsory vocational training are based. As a body equivalent to the specialist Royal Colleges, the College escapes the uneasiness that has at times pervaded relationships between them and the British Medical Association. The future strength of medicine in the National Health Service will depend chiefly on the development of a true consensus within the profession such as has not existed in the past. This is needed even more for the evolution of the best medical practice than for the profession's narrow, economic objectives.

There can be no doubt that the College will be needed, as medicine becomes increasingly subdivided into specialties, and general practice is established as the gatekeeper to the NHS. But it is not that alone. The general practitioner and the other professionals who work with him handle most of the episodes of illness or fear of illness which bring people to seek NHS help. People do not see themselves as using the NHS, so much as consulting their own personal physicians. If the NHS is to go farther, as it surely will, in a preventive role of trying to identify possible controllable or even removable illness or disability, it will be through general practice that that is secured. As the hospital specialties become narrower and more sharply defined, the position of the general practitioner as the selector of the occasion and the nature of the use of specialized services becomes even more important. As David Mechanic has pointed out, all countries already ration the use of health care in some way, according to need or affluence of users or the availability of resources. In some systems the affluent have the use of even more medical technology than they need, while the uninsured or the poor have less. In this uncertain situation we would have to invent the College for the future if we did not have it now.

General practice now is widely variable in quality. There must be variability in method and organization, as people differ so widely themselves. Nevertheless, the outcome for patients should be brought uniformly to as high a standard as can be achieved. That must be the primary aim of the College and it requires a commitment to education of the student, to vocational training of the qualified and to ongoing education of those already in practice. Since many others participate in complete health care it follows that there is an indirect concern with the way in which those others are trained – from practice receptionists to consultants in the regional specialties. With receptionists the concern is close; with health visitors, nurses and midwives it is less direct; with the techniques of pharmacy and ophthalmic optics it hardly exists, though there is mutual concern about organization of practices. It is questionable whether there is any field of medical practice in which some direct experience in general practice would be without benefit.

Study of methods and needs in practice must be a continuous process. Some of those needs are the result of biomedical scientific advance; some are the concomitants of general social change. Either will be the more readily absorbed into current usage if the individual special experience is generalized through the constant process of interchange within the College. Moreover, the existence of the regional faculties makes it easier to use the special local insight or progress which might pass unmarked in a body as centralized as are the other Royal Colleges. Their narrow concern with techniques and science too often blinds them to important social components of change. Many special reports of the Royal College of General Practitioners, symposium proceedings or Occasional Papers have helped members to a wider understanding, as has the quality of the College's *Journal* which is deservedly more widely read than other comparable publications. There has been much more activity of this kind in the College than in other Royal Colleges, largely because it has been undertaken as a component of a process of advance rather than as a firm, positive statement intended to be definitive for the time. It is important that this promoting rather than finalizing approach should continue. These comments are not critical of other Colleges, but merely emphasize different natures and situations.

The College is firmly established in the field of research because it offers an unique access to large numbers and continuous observation over long periods. Some of the earliest research was of a naturalistic kind, following in the tradition of Pickles of Aysgarth; but the College now has machinery of a far more sophisticated nature which is available to help its members with advice or resources. Some small studies come to the Scientific Foundation Board for support or to the Research Committee of Council for guidance; but so large a membership might be expected in future to yield a larger harvest.

The universities, other colleges and even the Medical Research Council have not yet appreciated how large a resource the Research Register of the College provides. It should be possible to encourage larger developments from this source. There are, for instance, many uncertainties about the needs which the rapidly growing number of old people will present in the remaining years of this century. There are also obvious requirements in the field of drug monitoring which can only be met through general practice.

One of the largest defects in the National Health Service is the failure to study the results of treatment of patients. Cochrane[1] and others have eulogized the controlled clinical trial as essential to monitoring the outcome of treatment. In much of the work of practice this kind of trial with mathematical studies of sharply definable outcomes such as death, or measurable parameters like blood pressure, would not be useful. The human outcome for the patient of a rather large investigation has to be measured in other terms. A recent attempt by Bunker, Barnes and Mosteller to put dollar values on such variables as pain, disability or survival is no better. Perhaps period of disability, at least for the employed, would be usable in some conditions, and relief of pain in others. Close evaluation may well require the elaboration of new methods such as some sociologists have attempted; even the fact of systematic scrutiny would help in itself, as McColl[2] has shown in the context of general surgery and Fry in general practice. Some general-practice groups are already doing this, especially those which use modern records systems. The College's work on records has been useful; but it needs to be pressed further, preferably in association with hospital improvements such as the problemoriented medical records system. There are some subjects, such as neonatal mortality, where district studies by hospital and community staff, jointly, are essential.

Research of this operational kind may not yield conclusions expressed in figures. Its most useful outcome may be at the district level in producing modification of service as well as of individual practice. That in turn may encourage generalization of any considerable result; but it is still in better realization of the generalist/specialist shared responsibility for health care that personal satisfaction and improved service is obtained.

The focal point in any health-care district should be the postgraduate centre. These centres have been a major College interest for nearly 20 years, but their working needs constant review. Success is not measured by head-counting or dignified occasions with formal orations. The centres should be the places where specialist and generalist knowledge is pooled and expanded – preferably in a multidisciplinary setting. There are some subjects, notably clinical pharmacology, in which the progress of knowledge is continuous to an extent that demands organized exposition. Breckenridge in Liverpool, Rawlins in Newcastle, Parish in Cardiff and others have attempted to organize this. As the Royal Commission has pointed out, pharmacists should be enabled to make a larger contribution in general practice and in hospital too – not as physicians *manqués*, but in their own professional capacity.

The College has so far approached health education somewhat gingerly. Yet primary and continuing care for a practice population is always expected to include some technical prophylactic interventions such as immunization. We pride ourselves on general practice as the field of the personal physician giving continuing care. It cannot be claimed that this is done effectively if opportunities of giving advice which would help prevent ill health are neglected or even deliberately eschewed. Some practitioners have become practised users of radio. The Health Education Council has held highly successful conferences of 50 or more doctors interested in participating. But it is common ground in health education that a health message is more credible and effective when it emanates from a known and respected source. Specifically a practitioner's advice on giving up smoking is known to be one of the most successful anti-smoking measures; equally it is reported that many general practitioners do not give that advice. Admittedly it would be difficult for the one-in-five-doctors who still smoke to be convincing; but it is inconceivable that that lamentably high proportion will continue. Meanwhile there are the other four. All doctors know that smoking is the largest, single, avoidable cause of premature death; and every general practitioner knows of one or two in his practice every year. But health promotion should not be seen in this narrow frame; it is well known that a health-promoting life style can greatly reduce ill health during life and prolong life expectancy. Advice on such a life style is not necessarily wilfully rejected by the individual – it may be presented to him at the wrong time when the social circumstances which facilitate it are absent. The general practitioner and the College can help in these situations.

All Colleges adopt some paraphernalia of pomp and exclusiveness. Some members have alleged that this College has copied too many of these attributes from the older bodies. While not accepting that, the possibility is certainly one against which the College must safeguard itself. Its real strength must reside in its regional faculties and especially in those regions where postgraduate development is active and preferably a chair of general practice exists. It is important that the College should maintain its countrywide base, even though that condemns its leaders to much travelling. Heavy demands will also be made for representative activity, but participation in the joint activities of Royal Colleges is essential. So far a National Institute or Academy of Medicine has failed to emerge from various suggestions of the need for it. As a result a single voice conveying a considered medical view or a commentary on the diversity is unobtainable. The British Medical Association has achieved some collation of views on the medicopolitical front, but it is not structured to deal with the main medical scientific issues. Until an Academy or a consortium of the Colleges is made effective, the College leadership must be involved in intercollegiate activities. There is thus a conflict of interest in a specialty whose real strength is peripheral but whose influence in the central councils of medicine may be decisive in avoiding the weakness which conflicting specialty influences might otherwise cause. It is upon the solution of that dilemma that the future of the College ultimately depends.

Reference has already been made to the educational activities of the College, but the emphasis of its work on undergraduate education must increase. There are still too many medical schools outside Scotland in which Departments of General Practice either do not exist or have not yet obtained Chairs. Ultimately the College must hope to see an adequate Department with a Chair in every medical school. The Jephcott Professorships have been used to help establish the need for improved teaching on primary care in a succession of schools. Given the funds, many would have established such Chairs by now. There are still some schools in which the value of undergraduate training in general practice is underestimated. The academic contribution may be thought trivial. There is also the risk that some academic departments which have been established become too far withdrawn into the academic role. The influence of the College is needed to guard against both these extremes. If general practice is to be taught – as it should be – the teaching must be based in a real-life practice situation and not an artificial clientele predominantly of people associated with the school. It is the social as much as the technical medical component of practice which the student needs.

In recent years some writers, such as Illich[3], have been sharply critical of the role of medicine in our society. Sociologists have often been critical of the human and community relationships of medical practice. Some practitioners have reacted against the non-scientific component of their work in relation to minor illness. It is often suggested that specially prepared nurses could undertake much of the work now considered medical at least as effectively as can doctors. This sort of difficulty is less likely to arise when a multidisciplinary team, providing primary care, in patterns such as Marsh and Kaim Caudle[4] have described, than in excessively technically orientated small practices. Where the team discharges fully the social as well as the technical components of health care there may be less tendency to enlarge practice populations. This is an area in which the College might well develop leadership provided it is able to carry the other professions with it. The emphasis is not wholly medical.

Finally, the College should concern itself increasingly with improvement of public relations in practices. The recent movement for patient committees in a few practices was mentioned favourably in the Royal Commission's Report[5]. This movement has had some help from the College and deserves more. Some Community Health Councils have shown great goodwill towards general practice; it is important that the College should help to develop that more widely. Primary health care will not again slip back into the condition once described as that of a 'cottage industry', and goodwill is most likely to be ensured by a conscious effort of the College to meet and satisfy public interest.

References

1. Cochrane, A. L. (1972). *Effectiveness and Efficiency*. (London: Nuffield Provincial Hospitals Trust)
2. McColl, I. (1979). Medical audit in British hospital practice. *Br. J. Hosp. Med.,* **22,** 485–486, 488–489
3. Illich, I. (1976). *Limits to Medicine. Medical Nemesis: the Expropriation of Health.* (Harmondsworth: Penguin)
4. Marsh, G. and Kaim-Caudle, P. (1976). *Team Care in General Practice.* (London: Croom Helm)
5. Royal Commission on the National Heath Service (1979). *Report.* (London: HMSO)

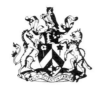

APPENDICES

---

1. HONORARY FELLOWS

W. J. H. M. BEATTIE, MD, FRCS, FRCOG
W. A. CONOLLY, MB, ChM, FRACGP
L. H. CORDERY, MB, ChB
H. M. SAXBY, *OBE, ED,* MB, FRACGP
Sir HARRY JEPHCOTT, *Bt.* MSc, HonDSc, FRIC, FPS
G. F. ABERCROMBIE, *VRD,* MD
G. O. BARBER, *OBE,* MB, BChir
D. M. HUGHES, BSc, MB, BChir
A. TALBOT ROGERS, CBE, MD, BS
SYLVIA G. DE L. CHAPMAN, MD, LM, DGO
Mrs THELMA GLYN HUGHES, MBE
The Rt Hon. LORD COHEN OF BIRKENHEAD, CH, MD, DSc, LLD, FRCP, HonFACP
The Rt Hon. LORD PLATT, MSc, MD, FRCP, HonFACP
R. J. F. H. PINSENT, *OBE,* MD
The Rt Hon. LORD AMULREE, *KBE,* MD, FRCP
Professor CHARLES M. FLEMING, *CBE,* MD, FRCP(Ed)
J. C. CAMERON, *CBE, TD,* MB, ChB
DAME ANNIS GILLIE, *DBE,* MB, BS, HonMD(Ed), FRCP
Professor J. C. VAN ES, MD
D. C. BOWIE, *OBE,* MB, ChB, FRCS(Ed)
J. J. ZACK, MD, FCFPG
Mrs EILEEN PHILLIPS
Sir JOHN BIGGART, *CBE,* MD, FRCP
C. W. CLAYSON, *CBE,* MD, DPH, FRCP
Professor C. R. LOWE, MD, PhD, MRCP, FFCM, DPH
H. R. H. THE PRINCE PHILIP, Duke of Edinburgh, *KG, KT*
W. A. FALK, MD, FCFPC
B. HALLIDAY, MD, FCFPC
LADY WOLFSON
Sir GEORGE GODBER, *GCB,* DM(Oxon), FRCP, DPH

255

Professor A. SMITH
Professor H. V. WARREN
Sir JOHN REVANS, *CBE*, LLD, FRCP, DCH
HILTON S. CLARKE
ANCRUM F. EVANS, *TD*, FCA
JOHN W. MAYO

2. HONORARY CHAPLAIN TO THE COLLEGE

The Rt Rev. GEORGE E. REINDORP, MA, DD, Bishop of Guildford. After 1973 The Lord Bishop of Salisbury

3. HONORARY SECRETARIES OF COUNCIL

1953   JOHN H. HUNT
1966   BASIL C. S. SLATER
1971   DONALD H. IRVINE

4. HONORARY TREASURERS OF THE COLLEGE

1953   H. L. GLYN HUGHES
1964   STUART J. CARNE

5. JAMES MACKENZIE LECTURES

1. Pickles, W. N. (1955). Epidemiology in the Yorkshire dales. *Practitioner*, **174**, 76–87
2. Barber, G. O. (1956). Medical education and the general practitioner. *Practitioner*, **176**, 66–78
3. Grant, I. D. (1957). Our heritage and our future. *Practitioner*, **178**, 85–97. *Research Newsletter, NS.4*, 7–23
4. Hughes, D. M. (1958). Twenty-five years in country practice. *Practitioner*, **180**, 93–105; *J. Coll. Gen. Practit.*, **1**, 5–22
5. Abercrombie, G. F. (1959). The art of consultation. *Practitioner*, **182**, 84–95; *J. Coll. Gen. Practit.*, **2**, 5–21
6. Jones, J. A. Ll. Vaughan. (1960). The general practitioner and industrial health. *Practitioner*, **184**, 93–102; *J. Coll. Gen. Practit.*, **3**, 9–32
7. Batten, L. W. (1961). The Medical Adviser. *Practitioner*, **186**, 102–112; *J. Coll. Gen. Practit.*, **4**, 5–18
8. Gillie, A. C. (1962). James Mackenzie and General Practice to-day. *Practitioner*, **188**, 94–107; *J. Coll. Gen. Practit.*, **5**, 5–21
9. Pinsent, R. J. F. H. (1963). James Mackenzie and research to-morrow. *Practitioner*, **190**, 114–126; *J. Coll. Gen. Practit.*, **6**, 5–19
10. Henderson, J. M. (1964). Looking back to Mackenzie. *Practitioner*, **192**, 128–140; *J. Coll. Gen. Practit.*, **7**, 9–23
11. Scott, R. (1965). Medicine in society. *Practitioner*, **194**, 3–16; *J. Coll. Gen. Practit.*, **9**, 3–16
12. McConaghey, R. M. S. (1966). Medical practice in the days of Mackenzie. *Practitioner*, **196**, 147–160; *J. Coll. Gen. Practit.*, **11**, 2–20
13. Watson, G. I. (1967). Learning and teaching by family doctors. *Practitioner*, **198**, 142–155; *J. Coll. Gen. Practit.*, **3**, 3–21
14. Gibson, R. (1968). Lucerna Pedibus Meis. *J. R. Coll. Gen. Practit.*, **15**, 3–22
15. Amulree, Lord (1969). James Mackenzie and the future of medicine. *Practitioner*, **202**, 152–162; *J. R. Coll. Gen. Practit.*, **17**, 3–11

16. Hodgkin, G. K. (1970). Behaviour – The community and the general practitioner. *Practitioner*, **204**, 177–184; *J. R. Coll. Gen. Practit.*, **19**, 5–11
17. Kuenssberg, E. V. (1971). General practice through the looking-glass. *Practitioner*, **206**, 129–145; *J. R. Coll. Gen. Practit.*, **21**, 3–16
18. Crombie, D. L. (1972). 'Cum scientia caritas'. *Practitioner*, **208**, 146–159; *J. R. Coll. Gen. Practit.*, **22**, 7–17
19. Hunt, J. H. (1973). The Foundation of a College. The conception, birth and early days of the College of General Practitioners. *Practitioner*, **210**, 144–161; *J. R. Coll. Gen. Practit.*, **23**, 5–20
20. Stevens, J. (1974). Brief encounter. *Practitioner*, **212**, 83–102; *J. R. Coll. Gen. Practit.*, **24**, 5–22
21. McCormick, J. (1975). Fifty years of progress. *Practitioner*, **214**, 87–98; *J. R. Coll. Gen. Practit.*, **25**, 9–19
22. Stone, M. C. (1976). The most alluring of occupations. *Practitioner*, **216**, 77–89; *J. R. Coll. Gen. Practit.*, **26**, 7–16
23. Fry, J. (1977). Common sense and uncommon sensibility. *Practitioner*, **218**, 106–118; *J. R. Coll. Gen. Practit.*, **27**, 9–17
24. Gray, D. J. P. (1978). Feeling at home. *Practitioner*, **220**, 131–139, 145; *J. R. Coll. Gen. Practit.*, **28**, 6–17

6. WILLIAM PICKLES LECTURES

1. Byrne, P. S. (1968) The passing of the 'eight' train. *J. R. Coll. Gen. Practit.*, **15**, 409–427
2. Horder, J. (1969). Education after the Royal Commission. *J. R. Coll. Gen. Practit.*, **18**, 9–21
3. Gardner, W. S. (1970). Training to be a doctor. *J. R. Coll. Gen. Practit.*, **19**, 319–330
4. McKnight, J. E. (1971). The art so long to learn. *J. R. Coll. Gen. Practit.*, **21**, 315–324
5. Maybin, R. P. (1972). Health centres and the family doctor. *J. R. Coll. Gen. Practit.*, **22**, 365–375
6. Swift, G. (1973). Education for responsibility. *J. R. Coll. Gen. Practit.*, **23**, 389–399
7. Marinker, M. (1974). Medical education and human values. *J. R. Coll. Gen. Practit.*, **24**, 445–462
8. Irvine, D. (1975). 1984, The quiet revolution. *J. R. Coll. Gen. Practit.*, **25**, 399–407
9. Knox, J. D. E. (1976). Peter Piper's peck. *J. R. Coll. Gen. Practit.*, **26**, 476–484
10. Parry, K. M. (1977). Community practice. *J. R. Coll. Gen. Practit.*, **27**, 327–333

7. FOUNDATION COUNCIL AWARDS

1955	R. J. MINNITT
1961	W. N. PICKLES
1963	W. H. BRADLEY
1964	J. C. GRAVES and
	VALERIE GRAVES
1967	E. V. KUENSSBERG
1968	M. BALINT
1971	B. CARDEW
1972	K. C. EASTON
1973	D. I. RICE
1975	S. J. CARNE

8. George Abercrombie Awards

1970   R. M. S. McConaghey
1973   W. A. R. Thomson
1975   Professor A. Mair

9. Fraser Rose Gold Medalists

1972   S. L. Barley
1973   A. W. Prince
1974   M. Faulkner
1975   A. Y. Ewing
1976   C. R. Hartshorn

10. John Hunt Fellow

1974   J. P. Horder

11. Honorary Registrar

1953   Sylvia G. De L. Chapman

12. Administrative Secretaries

1955   Commander A. E. P. Doran
1965   Eileen Phillips
1971   James Wood

13. College Solicitors

Linklaters & Paines, Barrington House, Gresham Street, London, EC2

14. College Auditors

Ancrum Evans, Rutherfords, 8 Eccleston Square, London, SW1

15. College Publications

Reports from General Practice

1965   No. 1   *Special Vocational Training for General Practice*
1965   No. 2   *Present State and Future Needs – first edition*
1965   *No. 3*   *Additional Payments for Wide Experience and Notable Service in General Practice: an outline scheme*
1966   No. 4   *General Practice in the New Towns of Britain*, by J. B. Dillane
1966   No. 5   *Evidence of the College of General Practitioners to the Royal Commission on Medical Education*
1967   No. 6   *The Implementation of Vocational Training*
1967   No. 7   *Education in Psychology and Psychiatry*
1968   No. 8   *General Practice in South-West England*
1968   No. 9   *Obstetrics in General Practice*

1968 No.10 *The Practice Nurse*
1969 No.11 *General Practice Teaching of Undergraduates in British Medical Schools*, by C. M. Harris
1970 No.12 *A Study of General Practitioners' Workload in South Wales 1965–1966* by W. O. Williams
1970 No.13 *Present State and Future Needs of General Practice* – second edition
1971 No.14 *The Future General Practitioner. Part 1. Problems of organizing his training*
1972 No.15 *Teaching Practices*, by Donald Irvine
1973 No.16 *Present State and Future Needs* – third edition
1976 No.17 *The Assessment of Vocational Training for General Practice*, by J. Freeman and B. S. Byrne

Journal Supplements

1956 *Conference on General Practitioner Obstetrics*
1956 *The Complications of Measles*
1957 *An Obstetric Survey*
1958 *The Problems of Stress in General Practice*
1958 *On Undergraduate Education and the General Practitioner*
1959 *Memorandum for the Guidance of Trainers*
1961 *Accident Management*
1961 *Emotional Disorders in General Practice*
1962 *A Guide to Research in General Practice*
1962 *The First Year of Life*
1963 *The Family Doctor and the Care of the Aged*
1963 *Nutrition in General Practice*
1963 *Arthritis in General Practice*
1963 *Migraine*
1964 *The Hazards of Middle Age*
1964 *Rehabilitation*
1964 *The Aetiology of Congenital Anomalies*
1964 *Forensic Medicine*, by A. J. Laidlaw and K. W. Cross
1965 *The Art and the Science of General Practice*
1965 *Problems of Sex in General Practice*
1965 *Antibiotics in Clinical Practice*
1966 *The Early Stages of Chronic Bronchitis*
1966 *Preventive Medicine and General Practice*
1966 *The Quality of Medical Care*
1966 *Health in a Changing Environment*
1967 *Clinical Problems of Practice*
1967 *Anaemia in General Practice*
1967 *The Art of Listening*
1967 *Group Practice, Ancillary Help and Government Controls*, by M. Hutchinson

1967   *Early Diagnosis*
1967   *The Medical and Social Problems of an Immigrant Population*
1968   *The Age of Discretion*
1968   *The Early Detection of Imported and Endemic Disease*
1969   *Society and its General Practitioners*
1969   *Adolescence and its Problems*
1969   *Psychiatry in General Practice*
1969   *The Sixth and Seventh Ages of Man*
1969   *Rheumatology in General Practice*
1969   *Communicable Diseases*
1970   *Man, Milieu and Malady*
1970   *The Management of Staff in General Practice*
1970   *A Future in General Practice*
1970   *Group Practice*
1971   *Survey of General Practitioners' Care of their Patients in the Hospital Service*
1971   *Transport Services in General Practice*
1971   *The Prescribing of Psychotropic Drugs*, by Peter A. Parish
1972   *General Practitioners and Abortion*
1972   *General Practitioners and Contraception in 1970–71*
1972   *General Practice in the London Borough of Camden*
1972   *The Renaissance of General Practice*, by John H. Hunt
1973   *University Department of General Practice and the Undergraduate Teaching of General Practice in the United Kingdom in 1972*, by P. S. Byrne
1973   *The Medical Use of Psychotropic Drugs*
1973   *A General Practice Glossary*, second edition by Research Unit of Royal College of General Practitioners
1974   *The Hostile Environment of Man*
1974   *A Visit to Australia and the Far East*, by George Swift
1976   *Prescribing in General Practice*

Occasional Papers

1976	No. 1	*An International Classification of the Health Problems of Primary Care*	The World Organization of National Colleges, Academies and Academic Associations of General Practitioners/Family Physicians
1976	No. 2	*An Opportunity to Learn*	E. V. Kuenssberg
1976	No. 3	*Trends in National Morbidity*	Royal College of General Practitioners
1977	No. 4	*A System of Training for General Practice* – first edition (second edition 1979)	D. J. Pereira Gray

Miscellaneous

1956	*Report on Medical Manpower*
1958	*Epidemic Winter Vomiting*
1958 –	*Morbidity Statistics from General Practice. Studies on Medical and*
1962	*Population Subjects.* No. 14 Vol. 1 by W. P. D. Logan and A. A. Cushion; Vol. 2 by W. P. D. Logan; Vol. 3 by College of General Practitioners
1959	*Coronary Artery Disease in General Practice*
1960	*Chronic Bronchitis in General Practice*
1961	*Obstetrics in General Practice*
1963	*Report of a Survey of General Practitioner Hospital Beds*
1963	*Guidance for Students Visiting a General Practitioner*
1965	*General Practice Tomorrow (Report of a Clinical Meeting)*
1966	*Medical History and the General Practitioner*
1967	*Design Guide for Medical Group Practice*
1967	*Family Health Care – The Team*
1972	*The Future General Practitioner – Learning and Teaching*
1973	*Sir James Mackenzie (Biography)*

INDEX